Manual of
Mysteries of Infertility Unravelled

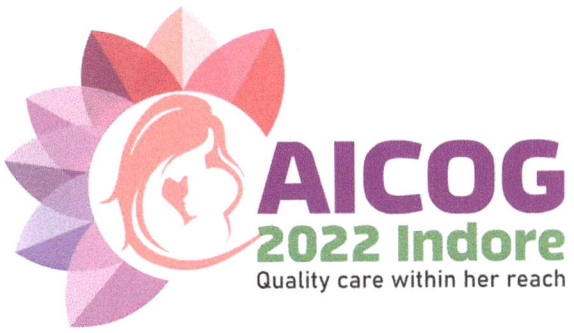

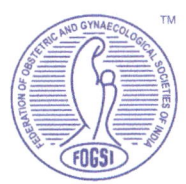 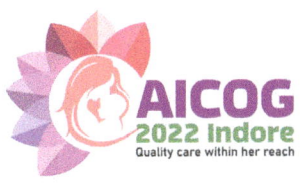 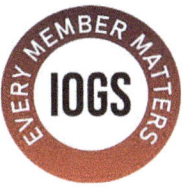 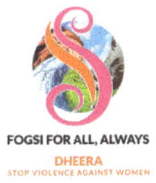

64th All India Congress of Obstetrics and Gynaecology
04–08 April 2022

Manual of
Mysteries of Infertility Unravelled

Editors

Mangla Kawade MBBS MD (Obs & Gyne)
Consultant Gynecologist and Fertility Specialist, Bhopal
Assistant Professor
Chirayu Medical College and Hospital
Bhopal, Madhya Pradesh, India

Shefali Jain MBBS MS (Obs & Gyne)
Director
Asian Institute of Infertility Management
Indore, Madhya Pradesh, India

Co-Editor

Shweta Kaul Jha MS FNB (Reproductive Medicine)
Director
ANAMAYA—Centre for Eye and IVF Care
Indore, Madhya Pradesh, India

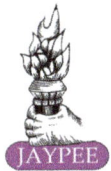

JAYPEE BROTHERS MEDICAL PUBLISHERS
The Health Sciences Publisher
New Delhi | London

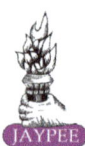 **Jaypee Brothers Medical Publishers (P) Ltd**

Headquarters
Jaypee Brothers Medical Publishers (P) Ltd
EMCA House, 23/23-B
Ansari Road, Daryaganj
New Delhi 110 002, India
Landline: +91-11-23272143, +91-11-23272703
+91-11-23282021, +91-11-23245672
Email: jaypee@jaypeebrothers.com

Corporate Office
Jaypee Brothers Medical Publishers (P) Ltd
4838/24, Ansari Road, Daryaganj
New Delhi 110 002, India
Phone: +91-11-43574357
Fax: +91-11-43574314
Email: jaypee@jaypeebrothers.com

Overseas Office
JP Medical Ltd
83 Victoria Street, London
SW1H 0HW (UK)
Phone: +44 20 3170 8910
Fax: +44 (0)20 3008 6180
Email: info@jpmedpub.com

Website: www.jaypeebrothers.com
Website: www.jaypeedigital.com

© 2022, Jaypee Brothers Medical Publishers

The views and opinions expressed in this book are solely those of the original contributor(s)/author(s) and do not necessarily represent those of editor(s) of the book.

All rights reserved. No part of this publication may be reproduced, stored or transmitted in any form or by any means, electronic, mechanical, photocopying, recording or otherwise, without the prior permission in writing of the publishers.

All brand names and product names used in this book are trade names, service marks, trademarks or registered trademarks of their respective owners. The publisher is not associated with any product or vendor mentioned in this book.

Medical knowledge and practice change constantly. This book is designed to provide accurate, authoritative information about the subject matter in question. However, readers are advised to check the most current information available on procedures included and check information from the manufacturer of each product to be administered, to verify the recommended dose, formula, method and duration of administration, adverse effects and contraindications. It is the responsibility of the practitioner to take all appropriate safety precautions. Neither the publisher nor the author(s)/editor(s) assume any liability for any injury and/or damage to persons or property arising from or related to use of material in this book.

This book is sold on the understanding that the publisher is not engaged in providing professional medical services. If such advice or services are required, the services of a competent medical professional should be sought.

Every effort has been made where necessary to contact holders of copyright to obtain permission to reproduce copyright material. If any have been inadvertently overlooked, the publisher will be pleased to make the necessary arrangements at the first opportunity. The **CD/DVD-ROM** (if any) provided in the sealed envelope with this book is complimentary and free of cost. **Not meant for sale**.

Inquiries for bulk sales may be solicited at: jaypee@jaypeebrothers.com

Manual of Mysteries of Infertility Unravelled

First Edition: **2022**

ISBN: 978-93-5465-627-9

Dedicated to
*All women aspiring to be
mother's against all odds!! against all logics!!*

Contributors

Atishay Jain MBBS MS FMAS DRMS
Director and Consultant
Asian Institute of Infertility
Management and
Dr Shefali Jain Test Tube Baby Centre
Indore, Madhya Pradesh, India

Kanthi Bansal MD DGO FICOG
Director
Safal Fertility Foundation
Ahmedabad, Gujarat, India

Keshav Malhotra MD
Lab Director
Rainbow IVF
Agra, Uttar Pradesh, India

Mangla Kawade MBBS MD (Obs & Gyne)
Consultant Gynecologist and Fertility
Specialist, Bhopal
Assistant Professor
Chirayu Medical College and Hospital
Bhopal, Madhya Pradesh, India

Manjiri Valsangkar MS (Obs & Gyne)
Diploma in Gynec Endoscopy Germany
Director
Bhide Hospital and IVF Centre
Pune, Maharashtra, India

Monica Singh MD DNB FMAS FICOG
Consultant Reproductive Medicine
Bhopal Fertility and Endoscopy Centre
Associate Professor
LN Medical College and JK Hospital
Bhopal, Madhya Pradesh, India
Vice President, Bhopal Obstetric and
Gynaecological Society

Niket Patel MD DMAS FMAS
Medical Director
Akanksha Hospital
Anand, Gujarat, India

Priya Bhave Chittawar MS
Consultant Reproductive Medicine
Bansal Hospital
Bhopal, Madhya Pradesh, India

Parasuram Gopinath MS
Senior Consultant and Scientific
Director
CIMAR Fertility Centre
A Unit of Edappal Hospitals Pvt Ltd
Kochi, Kerala, India

Sayali Kandari Provide degree
Embryology Laboratory Director and
Clinical Research Head
Senior Consultant Onsite/Offsite
Laboratory Director
Cellsure Biotech Research Centre
Thane, Maharashtra, India

Shefali Jain MBBS MS (Obs & Gyne)
Director
Asian Institute of Infertility
Management
Indore, Madhya Pradesh, India

Shivani Joshi DRM MS (Obs & Gyne)
Total Fertility Solutions
IVF Centre
Indore, Madhya Pradesh, India

Shreyas Padgaonkar MD DGO DNB
Director
Shreyas Fertility Centre
Mumbai, Maharashtra, India

Shweta Kaul Jha MS FNB (Reproductive Medicine)
Director
ANAMAYA—Centre for Eye and IVF Care
Indore, Madhya Pradesh, India

Sunita Arora MD FICOG FICS
Senior Consultant
Bloom IVF Centre
Fortis La Femme Hospital
New Delhi, India

Teena Gupta MS (Obs & Gyne) Diploma in IVF and Reprod Med Dip in Gyne Endoscopy
Gynecologist
Ashapunj Fertility and Gynaecology Centre
Bhopal, Madhya Pradesh, India

Message

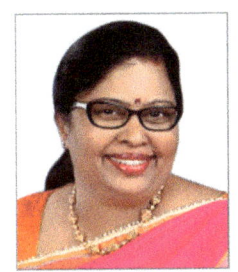 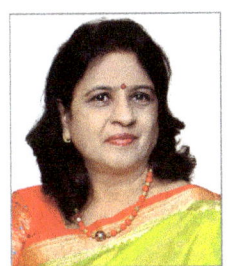

S Shantha Kumari
President, FOGSI

Madhuri Patel
Secretary General, FOGSI

Dear delegates
Dil se Namaste
Warm greetings!

On behalf of the organizing committee, I would like to welcome you all to our prestigious national conference—AICOG 2022.

This is being held after a gap of 2 long years. Long because of the uncertainties, hitherto unknown unprecedented road-blocks created by the scourge of the humanity COVID-19.

We are aware of the hard work and dedication of the Indore team. The way they have kept up their spirits is commendable.

As we move ahead in our path of scientific advances, we must ensure that it reaches out to the masses. Hence the theme of the conference "Quality Care within her Reach."

These workshops have been planned meticulously for you all to feast upon and enrich yourself with additional knowledge.

It has always been the endeavor of FOGSI to strive to impart knowledge with camaraderie and bonhomie, and both of us, wish you the very best.

Message from Organizing Committee

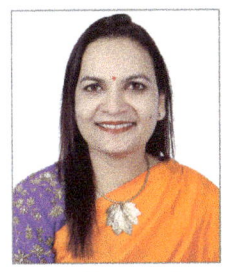
Asha Baxi
Organizing President

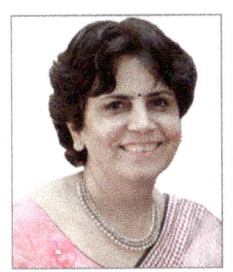
Kawita Bapat
Organizing Secretary

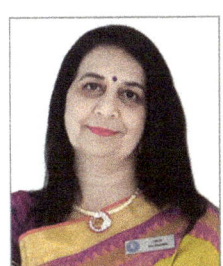
Archana Baser
Organizing Secretary

Dear All
Pranam, Namaste, and Swagatam
Welcome and Warm Greetings!

On behalf of the organizing committee, it gives us immense happiness to heartily welcome each one of you, to this revered prestigious National Conference of AICOG 2022.

Madhya Pradesh is the heart of India, and Indore being its 'Dil' become the warmest and cleanest place to welcome you all.

We as a team, will try our best, that you always have memories to cherish forever of this conference.

The Ob/Gyn fraternity of the whole of Madhya Pradesh, stands with solidarity to ensure you have an academic feast, to titillate/stimulate your brain.

The course of planning of AICOG 2022, was a tough one. We were always swinging with the pendulum of the time, very unsure of the feasibility of conference. The waxing and waning of COVID, made our preparations reach either acme or nadir.

Despite the hurdles, we are bound to enthrall you with a scientific bonanza rolled out. Scientific advances never stop with any pandemic or calamity.

We wish that you keep abreast of all the latest advances, be it in the management of the dreaded COVID in pregnancy, ART, vaginal surgeries, oncology, endoscopy, cosmetic and uro-gynecology, or ultrasound and fetal medicine.

After great deliberation, discussion and brainstorming, we finalized 8 Pre-congress Workshops on 9th January 2022; with live demonstrations, video presentations, interactive teachings and the thrills of drills, to ensure that you go back enriched and enthralled.

Youngsters have a comprehensive package of Obstetrics in the "Beginners Delights" from 'foundation' to the 'crescendo' learning the finer nuances of the practice of Ob/Gyn.

The advances in medicine and the easy availability of the Internet knowledge, has lead to dwindling patient-doctor faith and increasing unfound conflicts. As a gynecologist, it is our moral responsibility to ensure not only the physical, but 'mental and emotional' health of the woman.

Thus we have a separate workshop addressing these medicolegal issues such as the latest amendment in the MTP Act, POCSO Act, VAW (Dheera) Act, examination of a survivor, apart from interactive sessions on actual cases. You can spruce up your knowledge with experts of the field.

The theme of the conference is "Quality Care within her Reach", and it is our utmost endeavor to enrich you with the ability to impart quality care with humanity and humility.

The workshops are chosen with extreme conscious efforts to meet the highest academic standards in a limited time, and I am confident that you shall enjoy the limited overs match hugely.

We are looking forward to welcoming you to the wonderful city of Malwa, Indore. The city known for its culture, hospitality, unique Cusine and of course the cleanliness.

So do join us, in this extravaganza of knowledge, to quench your academic thirst.

Preface

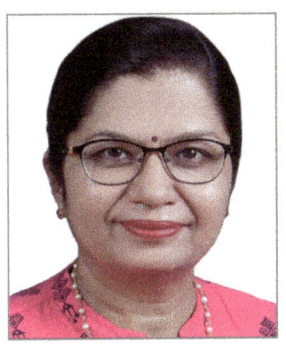

It gives us immense pleasure to welcome you all for 64th All India Congress of Obstetrics and Gynaecology (AICOG), 2022 to be held at Indore, Madhya Pradesh, cleanest city of India, fifth time in a row. We are thankful to management for entrusting us with this responsibility and we have put in our heart and soul to make it a success amidst this pandemic and unpredictable times. This workshop will enlighten us with latest aspects of assisted reproductive technology (ART), newer stimulation protocols, and advances in ART with artificial intelligence (AI). The variety of topics and seasoned speakers will make delegates get overall view of subject in simplified way. Along with great academics delegates can enjoy great historical and religious places in and around Indore along with best street food of country.

We wish you have a great time at the great infotainment event, first of this cadre post-pandemic.

Sumitra Yadav
Workshop Co-ordinator

Acknowledgments

We would like to acknowledge the extraordinary debt, we owe to the contributors for their precious time, knowledge, and experience they shared with us.

We feel a deep sense of gratitude towards editors, co-editors and organizing committee who worked in their full capacity for accomplishment of this manual.

Special thanks to those who gave their time to read or edit this manual and to all whose advice helped us in refining our ideas and approach throughout journey of creating this manual.

Contents

1. **Individualized Controlled Ovarian Stimulation** 1
   Monica Singh

2. **Freeze-all—Not for All** 3
   Shreyas Padgaonkar

3. **New Trends to Maximize Intrauterine Insemination Success Rates** 8
   Teena Gupta

4. **Thin Endometrial—Get Unstuck** 11
   Shefali Jain

5. **Optimizing Oocyte Retrieval and Embryo Transfer Technique: Tips and Tricks** 17
   Kanthi Bansal, Shweta Kaul Jha, Shivani Joshi

6. **Role of Laparoscopy Before IVF** 23
   Priya Bhave Chittawar

7. **Role of Adjuvants in Assisted Reproductive Techniques** 25
   Atishay Jain

8. **Ovarian Reserve Markers** 31
   Sunita Arora

9. **Premature Ovarian Ageing, Role of Platelet Rich Plasma and Stem Cells** 34
   Niket Patel

10. **Newer Stimulation Protocols: PPOS and DuoStim** 35
    Manjiri Valsangkar

11. **Vitrification: The Game-changer** 38
    Parasuram Gopinath

12. **Artificial Intelligence in IVF: A Need**.. 40
    Sayali Kandari, Keshav Malhotra

13. **Fertility in Women Beyond 35 Years**.. 45
    Mangla Kawade

14. **Salient Points of ART Bill, 2020**.. 49
    Shweta Kaul Jha

CHAPTER 1
Individualized Controlled Ovarian Stimulation

Monica Singh

The ideal ovarian stimulation regimen for IVF should have a low cancelation rate, minimize drug costs, have low risks and side effects, and maximize singleton pregnancy rates.

Individualization starts from an assessment before the start of in vitro fertilization (IVF) cycle of the ovarian reserve by antral follicle count (AFC), anti-Müllerian hormone (AMH), follicle-stimulating hormone (FSH), and age of the patient.

Once the patient is categorized as a hypo-/hyper- or normoresponder, the dose of gonadotropin is decided. The selection of dose is of paramount importance for optimal outcome of controlled ovarian stimulation (COS). This helps in explaining the prognosis and in appropriate counseling, and also ensures a safe COS. In women at high risk for ovarian stimulation, it is important to start with low doses and intensive monitoring. In case there are indications of hyperstimulation, the regime may be altered by decreasing dose or coasting. Many factors are interdependent, and hence, a careful selection of the type of ovarian stimulation will be the key factor in deciding the success of the same.

The main objective of individualization of treatment in IVF is to offer every couple the best treatment tailored to her own unique characteristics, thus maximizing the chances of pregnancy and eliminating the iatrogenic and avoidable risks resulting from ovarian stimulation. Personalization of treatment in IVF should be based on the prediction of ovarian response for every individual.

Evidence has demonstrated that AFC and AMH, the most sensitive markers of ovarian reserve identified to date, are ideal in planning personalized COS protocols. These sensitive markers permit prediction of the whole spectrum of ovarian response with reliable accuracy. Following the categorization of expected ovarian response to stimulation, clinicians can adopt tailored therapeutic strategies for each patient. Current scientific trend suggests the elective use of the gonadotropin-releasing hormone (GnRH) antagonist based regimen for hyper-responders, and probably also poor responders, as likely to be beneficial. The selection of the appropriate and individualized gonadotropin dose is also of paramount importance for effective COS and subsequent IVF outcomes.

Body mass index (BMI) and age of the patient have to be taken into consideration in order to tailor the exogenous gonadotropin dose, and adjuvant treatment should aim for high safety and a shortening of time to live birth.

Personalized IVF offers several benefits; it enables clinicians to give women more accurate information on their prognosis thus facilitating counseling especially in the cases of extremes of ovarian response. The deployment of therapeutic strategies based on selective use of GnRH analogs and the fine tuning of the gonadotropin dose on the basis of potential ovarian response in every single woman can allow for a safer and more effective IVF practice.

CHAPTER 2

Freeze-all—Not for All

Shreyas Padgaonkar

INTRODUCTION

Today almost all assisted reproductive technology (ART) treatment cycles depend on ovarian stimulation using different gonadotropin protocols with gonadotropin-releasing hormone (GnRH) analogs. As the number of treatment cycles have increased over years so are the concerns about incidence of ovarian hyperstimulation syndrome (OHSS) especially the severe form requiring hospitalization. It is reported that ~2% of the women undergoing in vitro fertilization (IVF) treatments suffer from severe form of OHSS. In early 2000s in the UK and Netherlands, 3 deaths were reported per 100,000 IVF cycles.[1,2] In view of this report, Devroey et al. proposed a concept of OHSS free clinic using a strategy of antagonist cycle with agonist trigger and freeze all for hyper-responders.[3] Documentation of equal effectiveness of antagonists compared to agonists and greatly improved outcomes of thawed vitrified embryos were the main reasons for such a suggestion. Over the years, new indications were for freeze-all strategy. Today there is a debate if freeze-all should be offered for all patients undergoing IVF.

We will look into different indications, current evidence regarding the advantages of freeze-all and potential risks involved.

ABSOLUTE INDICATIONS FOR FREEZE-ALL

1. Prevention of OHSS
2. Progesterone elevation
3. Preimplantation genetic testing for aneuploidies (PGT-A)/PGT cycles
4. Undiscovered pathological conditions
5. Slow developing blastocysts
6. Fertility preservation for cancer patients
7. Personalized embryo transfer (ET)
8. Random start or double stimulation protocol

Prevention of OHSS: Hyper-responders are at a high risk of OHSS, which is further increased in case the woman gets pregnant. Ovulation triggering with human chorionic gonadotropin (hCG) also adds to the risk of OHSS. Use of GnRH antagonists allows using GnRH agonists as a trigger instead of hCG. This strategy can almost eliminate the incidence of OHSS.[4] Suboptimal luteal phase resulting from GnRH agonist triggering is not a concern in freeze-all cycles.

Progesterone elevation: Progesterone rise before the trigger is associated with poor cycle outcome due to embryo endometrial asynchrony. These embryos can be frozen and transferred in synchronized cycle.[5]

PGTA/PGT cycles: Biopsied blastocysts need to be frozen, as the results of tests like comparative genome hybridization (CGH) are not available immediately.

Undiscovered pathological conditions: Evaluation of pelvis before IVF cycle is a norm, in spite of that some pathological conditions are diagnosed late in the stimulated cycles. Endometrial polyps, submucosal myoma, hydrosalpinx, thin endometrium, endometrial fluid accumulation, cervical stenosis can adversely affect the cycle outcome. Freezing all the embryos followed by surgical correction or optimization of endometrial preparation is preferred strategy.

Slow developing blastocysts: One of the reasons of lower implantation rates of day 6 blastocysts compared to day 5 is asynchrony with the endometrium. Healy et al.[6] documented comparable birth rates when frozen day 5 and day 6 blastocyst transferred.

Personalized ET after endometrial receptivity assay (ERA) for repeated implantation failures.

Random start or double stimulation protocol: Transfers in thaw cycles are warranted, as the endometrium is completely out of synch due to the nature of the stimulation protocols.

PROPOSED INDICATIONS FOR FREEZE-ALL

1. Higher pregnancy rates
2. Repeated IVF failure
3. Poor responders

Higher pregnancy rates: Stimulated cycles have high levels of estradiol. These supraphysiological levels are thought to be detrimental for embryo implantation. The endometrium may be advanced by 2–4 days in stimulated cycles as compared to natural cycles. Markers of implantation such as pinopodes and nucleolar channels also may appear early. Differences in gene expression are also proposed but the consequences of these differences on embryo implantation remain unknown.

Researchers have proposed that the freeze-all strategy improves IVF outcomes. The literature supporting these claims need to be scrutinized carefully before making freeze-all for every patient a clinical practice. In 2013, Roque et al.[7] claimed frozen embryo transfer (FET) compared to the fresh transfer improves the IVF outcome. They included three randomized controlled trials (RCTs) in their meta-analysis. One of the RCTs was later withdrawn for serious methodological flaws. The other two RCTs came from the same group of researchers, one of them included only high responders and the other normal responders both these trials had only 60–70 patients in each arm.

Studies looking at fresh versus frozen transfers in polycystic ovary syndrome (PCOS) women have documented higher live birth rates (LBRs) and lower pregnancy losses.[8]

In RCT involving normal responding women with day 3 transfer and vitrification, Vuong et al.[9] and Shi et al.[10] observed similar pregnancy rates and outcomes, whereas Wei et al.[11] after day 5 transfers observed better outcome in freeze-all cycles. All these trials used antagonist protocols. A recent RCT[12] involving unselected patients using long agonist protocol showed better results with fresh ET compared to FET. Meta-analysis conducted by Roque[13] in 2019 showed higher LBR in high responder and similar LBR in normal responders. A 2021 Cochrane review[14] observed no difference in cumulative live birth rate or ongoing pregnancy rate. Currently there is a lack of grade evidence in favor of freeze-all especially for live birth rates.

Repeated IVF failure: Impaired endometrial receptivity in fresh cycles is the hypothesis behind the use of freezes-all strategy for repeated IVF failures. There are very few studies and they are inconclusive[15,16] to support the use of this strategy.

Poor responders: In a study of 433 poor responders, no difference was observed between fresh and frozen ET.[17] A study by Acharya et al. documented better outcome in fresh ET in poor responders.[18]

SAFETY OF FREEZE-ALL STRATEGY (OBSTETRIC AND PERINATAL OUTCOME)

Health of infants born with FET has been a subject of scrutiny for some time. Data from the Swedish registry comparing 8,944 fresh and 2,348 thaw singleton pregnancies, reported higher incidence of large for gestational age (LGA) babies with higher perinatal morbidity and higher incidence of hypertensive disorders in pregnancy.[19] The CoNARTaS group data from the Scandinavian countries also documented increased risk of hypertensive disorders in pregnancies in ART pregnancies, which was more pronounced in FET cycles. In siblings, the risk was higher after FET cycles compared to the fresh cycles within the same mother.[20] A recent study analyzed 14,289 fresh and 11,098 frozen cycles after oocyte donation registered in the Society for Assisted Reproductive Technology Clinic Outcome Reporting System (SART CORS) database. This study reported a better good obstetric outcome (GBO), defined as a singleton, term, live birth with appropriate for gestational age birth weight, in fresh transferred compared to the FET.[21] RCTs, meta-analysis and Cochrane review for freeze-all strategies have raised concerns about the higher incidence of LGA babies and hypertensive disorders.[8,10,13,14] The effect of the day of transfer and the endometrial preparation used for FET may influence the outcomes of FETs.

RISKS INVOLVED IN FREEZING EMBRYOS

1. Cryo-damage
2. Toxicity of cryoprotectants
3. Potential equipment failure or liquid nitrogen supply failure
4. Breach of packaging and contamination in storage
5. Loss due to disaster or human errors

All of these can cause loss or reduction in the potential of embryos in storage.

OTHER CONSIDERATIONS

Couples want to minimize the time to pregnancy and freeze-all strategy lengthens this. It also adds the psychological burden of postponement of treatment.

The additional cost of embryo freezing and thaw ET may be 30% more than the fresh ET.

CONCLUSION

For patients with excess response to stimulation, freeze-all is an excellent strategy to prevent OHSS with high pregnancy rates. But every patient will not benefit from this approach. Also we need to keep in mind higher risk of adverse obstetric and neonatal outcome after FET. Currently, there are many RCTs underway to test this hypothesis which may throw more light on the use of freeze all for all.

The current evidence does not warrant use of a freeze-all for every patient.

REFERENCES

1. Bowyer L. Confidential Enquiry into Maternal and Child Health (CEMACH). Saving Mothers' Lives: reviewing maternal deaths to make motherhood safer 2003–2005. The Seventh Report of the Confidential Enquiries into Maternal Deaths in the UK. Obstet Med. 2008;1:54.
2. Braat DD, Schutte JM, Bernardus RE, et al. Maternal death related to IVF in the Netherlands 1984–2008. Hum Reprod. 2010;25:1782-6.
3. Devroey P, Nikolaos P. Polyzos, Blockeel C. An OHSS-Free Clinic by segmentation of IVF treatment. Hum Reprod. 2011;26:2593-7.
4. Melo M, Busso CE, Bellver J, Alama P, Garrido N, Meseguer M, et al. GnRH agonist versus recombinant HCG in an oocyte donation programme: a randomised, prospective, controlled, assessor-blind study. Reprod Biomed Online. 2009;19:486-92.
5. Venetis CA, Kolibianakis EM, Bosdou JK, et al. Progesterone elevation and probability of pregnancy after IVF: a systematic review and meta-analysis of over 60,000 cycles. Hum Reprod Update. 2013;19:433-57.

6. Healy MW, Yamasaki M, Patounakis G, Richter KS, Devine K, DeCherney AH, et al. The slow growing embryo and premature progesterone elevation: compounding factors for embryo-endometrial asynchrony. Hum Reprod. 2017;32:362-7.
7. Roque M, Lattes K, Serra S, Sol I, Geber S, Carreras R, et al. Fresh embryo transfer versus frozen embryo transfer in in vitro fertilization cycles: a systematic review and meta-analysis. Fertil Steril. 2013;99:156-62.
8. Chen Z-J, Shi Y, Sun Y, et al. Fresh versus frozen embryos for infertility in the polycystic ovary syndrome. N Engl J Med. 2016;375:523-33.
9. Vuong LT, Dang VQ, Ho TM, Huynh BG, Ha DT, Pham TD, et al. Freeze-all versus fresh embryo transfer in IVF/ICSI, a randomised controlled trial. Fertil Steril. 2016;106:e376.
10. Shi Y, Sun Y. Transfer of fresh versus frozen embryos in ovulatory women. N Engl J Med. 2018;378:126-36.
11. Wei D, Liu JY, Sun Y, Shi Y, Zhang B, Liu JQ, et al. Frozen versus fresh single blastocyst transfer in ovulatory women: a multicenter, randomised controlled trial. Lancet. 2019;393:1310-8.
12. Wong KM, van Wely M, Verhoeve HR, Kaaijk EM, Mol F, van der Veen F, et al. Transfer of fresh or frozen embryos: a randomised controlled trial. Hum Reprod. 2021;36:998-1006.
13. Roque M, Haahr T, Geber S, Esteves SC, Humaidan P. Fresh versus elective frozen embryo transfer in IVF/ICSI cycles: a systematic review and meta-analysis of reproductive outcomes. Hum Reprod Update. 2019;25:2-14.
14. Zaat T, Zagers M, Mol F, Goddijn M, van Wely M, Mastenbroek S. Fresh versus frozen embryo transfers in assisted reproduction. Cochrane Database Syst Rev. 2021;2(2):CD011184.
15. Magdi Y, El-Damen A, Fathi AM, Abdelaziz AM, Abd-Elfatah Youssef M, Abd-Allah AA, et al. Revisiting the management of recurrent implantation failure through freeze-all policy. Fertil Steril. 2017;108:72-7.
16. Bourdon M, Santulli P, Chen Y, Patrat C, Pocate-Cheriet K, Maignien C, et al. The deferred embryo transfer strategy seems not to be a good option after repeated IVF/ICSI cycle failures. Reprod Sci. 2019;26(9):1210-7.
17. Roque M, Valle M, Sampaio M, Geber S. Does freeze-all policy affect IVF outcome in poor ovarian responders? Ultrasound Obstet Gynecol. 2018;52:530-4.
18. Acharya KS, Acharya CR, Bishop K, Harris B, Raburn D, Muasher SJ. Freezing of all embryos in in vitro fertilization is beneficial in high responders, but not intermediate and low responders: an analysis of 82,935 cycles from the Society for Assisted Reproductive Technology registry. Fertil Steril. 2018;110:880-7.
19. Sazonova A, Källen K, Thurin-Kjellberg A, Wennerholm U, Bergh C. Obstetric outcome in singletons after in vitro fertilization with cryopreserved/thawed embryos. Hum Reprod. 2012;27:1343-50.
20. Opdahl S, Henningsen AA, Tiitinen A, Bergh C, Pinborg A, Romundstad PR, et al. Risk of hypertensive disorders in pregnancies following assisted reproductive technology: a cohort study from the CoNARTaS group. Hum Reprod. 2015;30:1724-31.
21. Roeca C, Johnson RL, Truong T, Carlson NE, Polotsky AJ. Birth outcomes are superior after transfer of fresh versus frozen embryos for donor oocyte recipients. Hum Reprod. 2020;35:2850-9.

CHAPTER 3

New Trends to Maximize Intrauterine Insemination Success Rates

Teena Gupta

▣ DEFINITION

A procedure to treat infertility in which processed semen is introduced into the uterine cavity with the rationale of increasing the density of energy-laden gametes at the time and the site of fertilization.

▣ INDICATIONS

- Mild male infertility
- Unexplained infertility
- Ovulatory dysfunction, polycystic ovarian syndrome (PCOS)
- Mild endometriosis grade 1 and 2
- Cervical factors
- Coital issues
- Immunological factors
- Infections such as HIV, HBsAg
- Donor sperm insemination
- Frozen samples when husband is not available or on antineoplastic treatment.

▣ STEPS OF IUI

- Evaluation and patient selection
- Ovarian stimulation
- Ovulation monitoring
- Semen preparation
- Insemination
- Luteal support

▣ SELECTION CRITERIA FOR GOOD SUCCESS RATES IN INTRAUTERINE INSEMINATION (IUI)

- Age of female < 35 years
- Duration of infertility < 5 years
- Good ovarian reserve based on serum anti-Müllerian hormone (AMH) and day 2 antral follicular count (AFC)
- Mild male factor infertility with total motile sperm count (TMSC) greater than 5 million per mL and normal sperms more than 4% (Equation

for calculation of TMSC = Sperm count in million per mL × Volume of ejaculate in mL × Percentage motility/100)
- Minimum one functional normal fallopian tube and no uterine factor

TIPS TO MAXIMIZE SUCCESS RATES

- Follow strict selection criteria of patients.
- Aim for two to three dominant follicles at maximum.
- In unexplained infertility following are the success rates:
  1. Natural cycle: 8%
  2. Clomiphene citrate (CC): 8–9%
  3. Letrozole: 12–14%
  4. Letrozole or CC plus gonadotropins: 20–22%
  5. Gonadotropins: 25%
- For gonadotrophin stimulation start with small dose 37.5–75 IU, step up by 37.5 IU, and take care response may be sudden and explosive once the threshold is crossed. According to Cochrane database systematic review, 2015 September, there is no difference in live birth rates between various gonadotropin preparations human menopausal gonadotrophin (hMG) versus follicle-stimulating hormone (FSH) and also among various types of preparations like urinary versus highly purified (HP) versus recombinant. Chronic low dose protocol is very effective in PCOS patients to decrease the incidence of multiple pregnancies and ovarian hyperstimulation syndrome (OHSS). In this protocol stimulation is started with 37.5–75 IU and is continued till 10–14 days before increasing the dose.
- Follicular monitoring with good ultrasound 2D, 3D and color Doppler improves the results.[1]
- Optimal pre-hCG (human chorionic gonadotropin) follicular parameters:
  1. Follicular diameter of minimum 16–17 mm and volume 3–7 cc
  2. Vascularity covering at least three-fourths of the follicular circumference
  3. Perifollicular resistance index (RI) 0.42–0.48
  4. Perifollicular PSV > 10 cm/s
  5. Follicular VI > 6, FI > 35
  6. Presence of cumulus oophorus
- Optimal pre-hCG endometrial parameters:
  1. Endometrial thickness minimum 6 mm, preferably 8 mm
  2. Grade A or B endometrium
  3. Vascularity in zone 3 or 4 covering more than 5 mm^2
  4. Endometrial RI 0.49–0.59 , PI 1.1–2.3
  5. Uterine artery PI < 3.2
  6. Endometrial volume > 3 cc
  7. Endometrial FI > 40, VFI > 20
- Abstinence interval of less than 3 days gives maximum pregnancy rate 14% and interval of more than 10 days pregnancy rate lower 3%.

- *Timing of IUI:* IUI gives best results when performed just before ovulation or within 10 hours of ovulation, so
  1. If serum LH > 10–12 mIU/mL or urine LH kit test positive do IUI 24 hours after LH surge, or
  2. If no LH surge does IUI 34–46 hours (average 38 hours) after ovulation trigger, or
  3. Double insemination at 12 and 36 hours in mild male factor infertility and donors' semen.
- No difference in outcome between semen preparation techniques swim-up or gradient techniques.
- Processed semen volume of 0.3–0.7 mL
- Insemination of sample 1–2 cm above the internal os
- Inseminate slowly over 3–5 minutes
- Wait for few seconds to prevent reflux
- Patient should lay supine for 10 minutes, no need of head low, restriction of routine activities, antibiotics and analgesics.
- Pregnancy rates in ultrasound-guided and blind insemination are similar.
- In difficult internal os negotiation, identify acute anteversion (then full the bladder) and acute retroversion (then empty the bladder) hold the cervix with Allies or tenaculum and give traction, in known cases do cervical dilatation on day 2 or 3 of menses.
- In cases of premature LH surge addition of GnRH antagonist along with gonadotropins may increase the pregnancy rates.
- *Role of adjuvants:* Insulin sensitizer drugs such as metformin or inositol may benefit in obese anovulatory PCOS. Other drugs with questionable efficacy are dexamethasone, estrogen, ecosprin, L-arginine, sildenafil, etc.
- *Luteal phase support:* Progesterone (oral or vaginal) increases the live birth rate in especially gonadotropins cycles.[2]

CONCLUSION

Evidence of financial, economics, and clinical considerations strongly favors IUI as a first-line treatment option for subfertility. IUI is a preferred method for ovulatory dysfunctions, unexplained infertility and mild male infertility. Superovulation along with a IUI increases the success rates.

REFERENCES

1. Panchal S, Nagori C. Can 3D PD be a better tool for assessing the pre HCG follicle and endoemntrium? A randomized study of 500 cases. Ultrasound Obstet Gynecol. 2006;28(4):504.
2. Hill MJ, Whitcomb BW, Lewis TD, Wu M, Terry N, DeCherney AH, et al. Progesterone luteal support after ovulation induction and intrauterine insemination: a systematic review and meta-analysis. Fertil Steril. 2013;100(5):1373-80.

CHAPTER 4

Thin Endometrial—Get Unstuck

Shefali Jain

■ INTRODUCTION

The endometrium is the most amazing and dynamic tissue in human body. It is considered to be complex, as it changes its pattern (structurally, biologically, endocrinologically, and functionally), with the cyclic variations and signals from steroid hormones in every phase of menstrual cycle.

The endometrium is involved with the final step of implantation, which not only requires a healthy embryo but a functioning as well as receptive endometrium.

Endometrial thickness (EMT) has been correlated with pregnancy and live birth rates, and has been considered as a prognostic factor for the final success of treatment.

In a case of subfertility, there may be defective endometrium with altered receptivity.

There could be various possible causes related to defective endometrium.
- Thin endometrium
- Endometrial polyp/persistently thick endometrium
- Fibroids
- Endometriosis
- Endometrial atrophy

■ DEFINITION AND INCIDENCE OF THIN ENDOMETRIUM

There is no agreement as to what thickness is considered to be normal or the common consensus on thin endometrium. The definition and cutoff for thin endometrium differs between studies, although most study use an EMT of <7 mm or <8 mm on the day of human chorionic gonadotropin (hCG) administration. The EMT of 4–5 mm does not exclude the possibility of pregnancy after embryo transfer (ET) but the chances of pregnancy are significantly low. The maximum pregnancy rate of EMT (9–14 mm) has been reported. To date, there is no common opinion in relation to the endometrium being too thick (>14 mm).

The incidence of thin endometrium <7 mm varies according to the chosen cutoff which is 1.49% in high responders and 2.5% in normal responders.

EVALUATION OF THIN ENDOMETRIUM

Many of potential risk factors have been identified from patient's history.
- Transvaginal sonography (TVS)
- Hysteroscopy—uterine cavity assessment by hysteroscopy or sonohysterogram may be performed in initial assessment of patient with thin endometrium to assess for pathological cause.

There are various ways to assess the endometrium but the simplest and noninvasive is an ultrasound in which we study the:
- Endometrial thickness
- Endometrial patterns
- Endometrial volume
- Doppler of uterine and sub-endometrial blood flow

Endometrial thickness is measured by TVS as the maximum distance between the echogenic interfaces of the myometrium and endometrium in sagittal plane of the uterus.

Endometrial pattern depicts the functional endometrium status. A three-layered endometrium showed a significantly higher pregnancy rates as compared with isoechogenic or hyperechogenic endometrium.

Endometrial volume has been suggested to play a role in predicting in vitro fertilization (IVF) outcomes. A volume of 3–5 mL in mid-cycle phase is optimum for good receptivity.

Color Doppler has also been suggested to play a role in predicting IVF outcomes. You try and serve intermediate blood flow has been assessed and classified into three zones according to blood flow patterns.

CLINICAL SIGNIFICANCE OF THIN ENDOMETRIUM

When thin ET detected during assisted reproductive technology (ART) cycle, the physician and patient face a decision whether or not to proceed with treatment. The patient should be informed about the possible solutions of the problem. These include the cycle continuation with potentially lower probability of pregnancy or discontinuation, with embryo cryopreservation and subsequent transfer of embryos in cryocycles.

There may be:
- Reduced chances of implantation
- Increased rates of miscarriages
- Higher incidence of ectopic pregnancies

WHY THIN ENDOMETRIUM REDUCES THE CHANCES OF SUCCESSFUL IMPLANTATION?

Immediately after ovulation the spiral arteries of the functional endometrium constrict and cause a reduction in blood flow to the functional layer.

The reduced blood flow decreases oxygen tension in implantation surface of the endometrial; this low oxygen environment appears to be more well coming to the embryo. This assumption is strengthened by the finding that embryo culture in vitro under low oxygen concentration show superior quality and outcome. This phenomenon is attributed to lower levels of free oxygen radicals and is now the standard practice in IVF laboratories.

It is still unclear why a thin endometrial lining reduces the chance of a successful implantation. A recent editorial written by Robert Casper provided a novel explanation to the poor outcome associated with a thin endometrium. According to this theory when an embryo is placed over a thin endometrium, it is closer the more vascularized stroma and therefore, exposed to a much higher oxygen tension. An alternative explanation suggests that the cause of a permanently thin endometrium is a dysfunction in the estrogen receptor that is involved both with endometrial proliferation and embryo implantation thereby impairing both endometrial proliferation and implantation.

CAUSES OF THIN ENDOMETRIUM

Implantation may a problem because of altered estrogen receptor's dysfunctions, oxygen tension theory, impaired angiogenesis and altered blood flow.

Common clinical conditions may be:
- Asherman's syndrome
- Previous intrauterine surgeries/D&C
- Infections postpartum endometritis, septic abortions
- Inflammatory—chronic endometritis
- Pelvic radiation
- Idiopathic—prolonged use off what is the pins or repeat the cycle so long if you citrate
- Hypogonadotropic hypogonadism, premature ovarian insufficiency, hyperandrogenic state
- Older women—5% in <40 years and 25% in >40 years. This is probably due to reduced endometrial vascularity.
- Controlled ovarian hyperstimulation (COH).

Endometrial compaction is an entity of defining endometrium which becomes thin in response to progesterone and results in optimal pregnancy outcomes in frozen embryo transfer (FET) cycles if it is found to be about 10%, ongoing pregnancy rate much higher. As compaction increases, chances of pregnancy become better.

THIN ENDOMETRIUM IN OVARIAN STIMULATION (NON-IVF) CYCLE

Thin endometrium is commonly encountered during ovarian stimulation (non-IVF) cycle. When patient undergoing OS have thin endometrium, clinician may consider whether to proceed with or cancel treatment cycle/ even IUI. They may be counseled that the effect of thin endometrium on pregnancy rates is still unclear. Thin endometrium may not impact pregnancy outcomes in OS treatment cycles evidence did not find a difference in EMT in patients who were pregnant versus those who were not.

Sometimes changing the stimulation medications are suggested but there is again insufficient evidence.

The recommended uses of adjuvants to improve EMT have not been proved.

THIN ENDOMETRIUM IN IVF (FRESH OR FROZEN CYCLES)

The impact of thin endometrium on IVF results have been studied extensively, although more data available on fresh treatment cycles.

In fresh-IVF embryo transfer cycles, patients with ET < 8 mm, there may be a negative impact on pregnancy and live birth rates. These patients should be offered elective cryopreservation of embryos and transfer in subsequent cycles.

In frozen IVF embryo transfer cycles, patients should be counseled that EMT < 7 mm has a negative impact on pregnancy and live birth rates.

For these patients with history of thin endometrium, in FET cycles, any specific protocol (natural or hormone replacement) for endometrial preparation may not be useful.

Methods of correction of thin endometrium:
- High dose of estrogen in the cycle of ovarian stimulation cycle or in FET cycle
- Drugs improving that circulation in the cycle of ovarian stimulation or a FET cycles
- Use of granulocyte colony-stimulating growth factor
- Autologous platelet rich plasma (PRP) infusion
- Endometrial scratching

TREATMENT OPTIONS

There are various treatment options to improve the EMT in women with thin endometrium.
- *Hormonal*:
  - Extended use of exogenous estrogens
  - Higher dose, longer duration, change route
  - HCG priming in the follicular phase 150 IU daily be D7 to D13
  - GnRH agonist during the luteal phase of OPU, ET
- *Growth factors:*
  - Growth hormone—tamoxifen

- *Vascular*:
  - Aspirin
  - L-arginine
  - Tocopherol with pentoxifylline
  - Vaginal sildenafil citrate
  - Electroacupuncture
  - Application of granulocyte colony-stimulating factor (G-CSF)
  - Using autologous PRP
  - Stem cell therapy

Aspirin

Aspirin has an antithrombotic and vasodilatory effect, and improves uterine and ovarian vascularization, but its effect in improving EMT is still controversial as no significant difference in EMT pregnancy or live birth rates.

L-arginine

Its use in the dose of 6 mg/day for women with their endometrium has been recommended. Nitric oxide (NO) synchronizes from L-arginine course relaxation of smooth muscles, by elevating the cyclic guanosine monophosphate (cGMP) levels. It has an effect on endometrial proliferation, thus providing an adequate environment for embryo adhesion and implantation.

Tocopherol with Pentoxifylline

Tocopherol (Vitamin E) has antioxidant properties. Vitamin E improves uterine vascularization and EMT by increasing VEGF expression. Studies showed that there is an increase in EMT but no significant difference in implantation and pregnancy rates.

Pentoxifylline has not only vasodilating, antiaggregant and anticoagulant properties but also anti-inflammatory and antifibrotic actions. It also antagonizes TNF-α production.

A combination of 400 mg pentoxifylline and 500 mg vitamin E twice daily for 6 months showed significant improvement in EMT.

All said and done these medications may be beneficial only in few cases but not in all cases of thin endometrium.

Sildenafil

It causes vasodilatation (relaxation of smooth muscles through a cGMP-mediated pathway). It augments the vasodilatory effects of NO on vascular smooth muscles by preventing the degradation of cGMP. It also improves endometrial arterial blood flow.

Many case series have reported the use of sildenafil for fresh or frozen IVF embryo transfers, with improvement in EMT but insufficient evidence to improve the pregnancy rates.

Granulocyte Colony-stimulating Factor

Granulocyte colony-stimulating factor is a glycoprotein that carries out both cytokine and growth factor activities. Intrauterine instillation of G-CSF produced successful thickening of the endometrium, in patients previously resistant to other therapies. However, some studies failed to show an improvement in pregnancy rate and implantation rate

Platelet-rich Plasma

Autologous PRP increased proliferation of not only cultured fibroblasts, but also of mesenchymal cells which are progenitors of different types of cells including endometrial cells. So, it is hypothesized that PRP stimulates cellular processes involved in endometrial regeneration. Chang et al. studies reported for the first time, an improvement in the EMT after intrauterine instillation of autologous PRP. Pregnancy also occurred in all these patients. Another study showed that PRP is effective in improving pregnancy outcome in recurrent implantation.

PRP is introduced into the uterine cavity with a Tomcat catheter (0.5–1 mL). If necessary PRP infusion can be performed one to two times more, the last infusion being 48 hours before embryo transfer. EMT can be reassessed 48–72 hours after the instillation. PRP can also be injected sub-endometrially and hysteroscopically.

Stem Cell Therapy

Endometrial stem or progenitor cells are found in the basalis and functionalis layers of the human endometrium. Stem cells as a source for regenerating different tissues are widely investigated. Research found out that human endometrial adult stem cells are able to generate human endometrium after transplantation in nonobese diabetic-severe combined immunodeficiency (NOD-SCID) mice renal capsules.

In a case of thin endometrium (3.6 mm) secondary to Asherman's syndrome and which was refractory to E2 treatment, autologous endometrial angiogenic stem cells were infused into the uterine cavity. This was followed by high dose of E2 valerate, aspirin 75 mg daily and four cycles of cyclical estrogen and progesterone therapy. EMT reached 7.1 mm.

■ CONCLUSION

Persistent thin endometrium is an infrequent but remains the most challenging disorder in reproductive medicine. No definite treatment has yet been established, and options are limited and are not problem specific. Currently minimal evidence to signify any improvement in pregnancy outcomes in patients with thin endometrium. Physician must balance the prognosis for patients if they proceed to treatment with thin endometrium or consider alternative treatments.

CHAPTER 5

Optimizing Oocyte Retrieval and Embryo Transfer Technique: Tips and Tricks

Kanthi Bansal, Shweta Kaul Jha, Shivani Joshi

■ TIPS AND TRICKS IN OOCYTE RETRIEVAL

Definition
Oocyte pick-up (OPU) is an ultrasound-guided technique in which oocytes are aspirated using a needle connected to a suction pump as per the European Society of Human Reproduction and Embryology (ESHRE) Consensus, 2019. There are different terms and abbreviations used in clinical practice such as oocyte retrieval, egg retrieval, oocyte collection, and follicle aspiration.

History
In 1983, the first transvaginal OPU was performed which was a major breakthrough. Other techniques such as laparoscopic or transabdominal pick-up were also developed but are rarely used.

Preparation
Prior to OPU, pelvic ultrasound, vaginal infection screening, patient medical history, information provision and informed consent have to be done. The patient is offered controlled ovarian stimulation (COS) with gonadotropins, either agonist or antagonist protocol. It is recommend scheduling the procedure at 36-hour interval between medical triggering and OPU, but intervals between 34 and 38 hours have been applied.

Patient Positioning
Although minimally invasive, these procedures need to be done in operation theaters (OTs) with all emergency drugs, gadgets, and competent anesthetist and team. Semilithotomy, lithotomy or sitting position on a comfortable gynecological table is preferred with buttocks at the edge of table.

Anesthesia
Short intravenous (IV) sedation or general anesthesia is preferred. IV fentanyl, propofol and midazolam are the most common medication used.

Ultrasound System

High-frequency transvaginal ultrasound transducer with the best quality real-time imaging system is used. Fit-in biopsy guide kits are available. Color Doppler study can help to detect vascular areas and visualize major vessels in proximity of ovary. 3D ultrasound which can exactly count on number and volume of follicles may help in safer performance but needs more studies in future.

Needle

Single-lumen needle of 17–18 G with echo-tip end is preferred. Double-lumen needles for flushing the follicle with media are available as well.

Lab and OT Preparation

Test tube warmer, heating blocks, and culture media for flushing are all kept at 37°. Each and every instrument has to be checked before OPU. The suction pressure of 100–140 mm Hg is considered safe for oocyte cumulus complex.

Technique

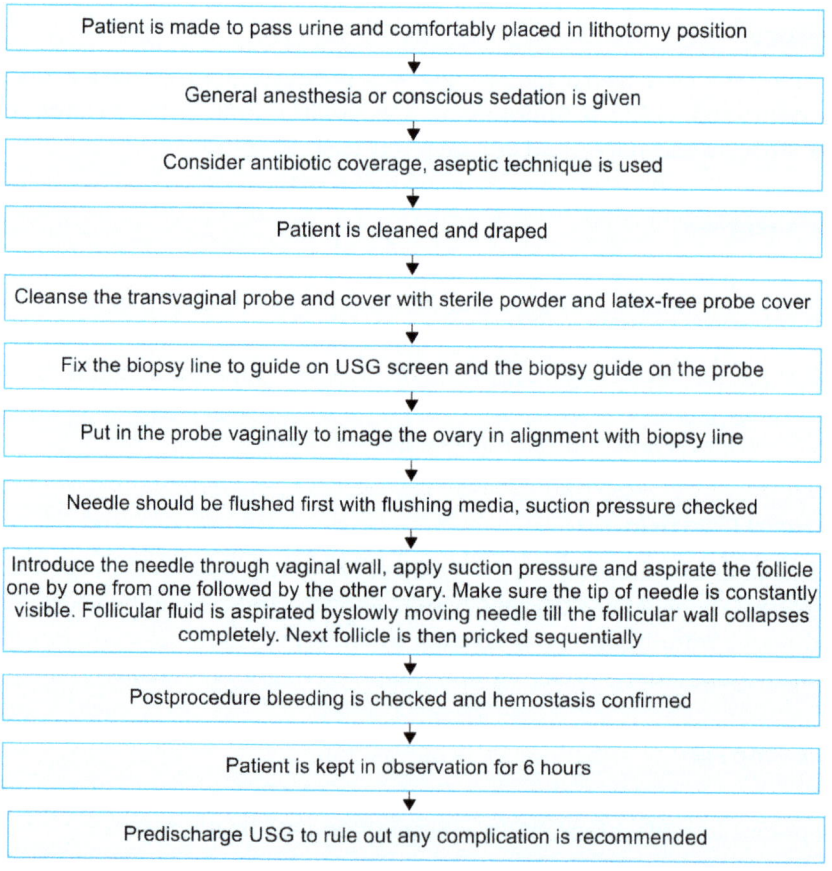

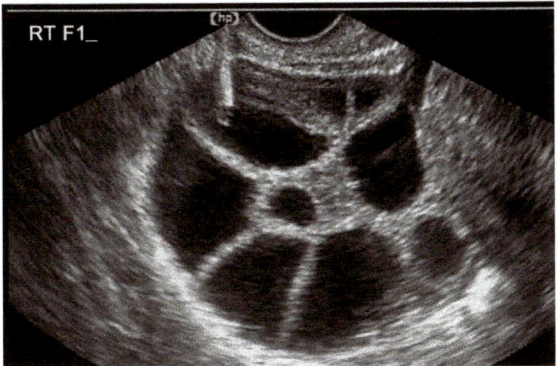

Fig. 1: Echogenic needle tip appreciated during ovum pick-up.

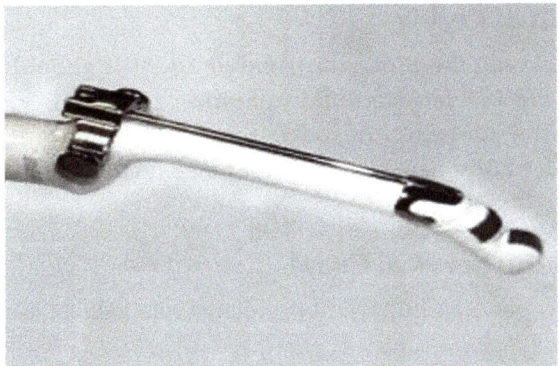

Fig. 2: Biopsy guide correctly placed over transvaginal USG probe.

Complications

The most common complications reported are vascular as internal pelvic bleeding, followed by pelvic infections and pelvic abscesses, injury to adjacent bladder and bowel. A systematic approach in performing OPU will ensure a low evidence of complications.

Conclusion

OPU is a low-risk surgical procedure but sometimes serious complications do occur. Therefore, the fine art of OPU has to be learnt by proper training and practice.

■ TIPS AND TRICKS IN EMBRYO TRANSFER

History

The world celebrated the first IVF baby birth in July, 1978. The present approach of transcervical embryo transfer evolved after multiple attempts of transfundal and transmyometrial approaches.

Preparation

Usually anesthesia is not required for this procedure. Partially full bladder is preferred for transabdominal USG-guided embryo transfer which is the most commonly used technique.

Patient Positioning

Patient is made to lie down in lithotomy or semilithotomy position with the hips placed at the edge of the gynecological table. It is believed that a full bladder could straighten the uterocervical angle during embryo transfer and facilitate access into the uterine cavity with a soft catheter.

The pitfall of an overfilled bladder, however, is patient discomfort, which arguably could increase uterine contractility.

Visualization of Cervix

Before commencing the procedure, patient identity should be confirmed according to the IVF lab standard operating protocols. Visualization of the cervix with a speculum in the setting of embryo transfer should be performed with utmost care to avoid initiating pain that could trigger uterine contractions.

Cleaning of the Cervical Canal

Cervical mucus plays an important protective role against ascending bacterial infection.

However, during IVF, an excessive amount of mucus (from the effect of progesterone) may interfere with embryo transfer by blocking the tip of the catheter or hindering embryo expulsion into the right place in the endometrial cavity.

So initially cervical mucus can be removed and cervical canal flushed with media, completely depending on clinician choice.

Role of Ultrasound Scan in Embryo Transfer

Transabdominal ultrasound-guided embryo transfer was first reported in 1985. Adequately full bladder, i.e., the uterine fundus should be completely visible is known to improve visualization of catheter advancement and tip placement thus improve the pregnancy rate. Use of ultrasound-guided embryo transfer has the potential benefit of visualization of the tip of the catheter allowing confirmation that the placement of the embryos has occurred beyond the internal os into the "optimal" place in the uterine cavity.

Mock Transfer

Mock transfer is a trial transfer technique like a rehearsal before actual procedure. It can be done at the time of starting the stimulation or at the time of oocyte retrieval or before actual embryo transfer.

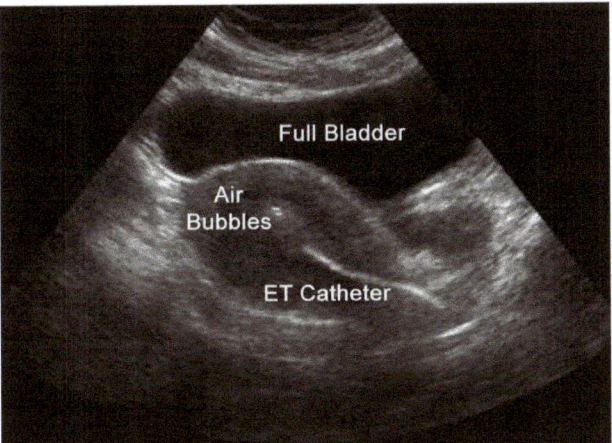

Fig. 3: Echogenic catheter used to place embryos in uterine cavity, 1–1.5 cm below fundus.

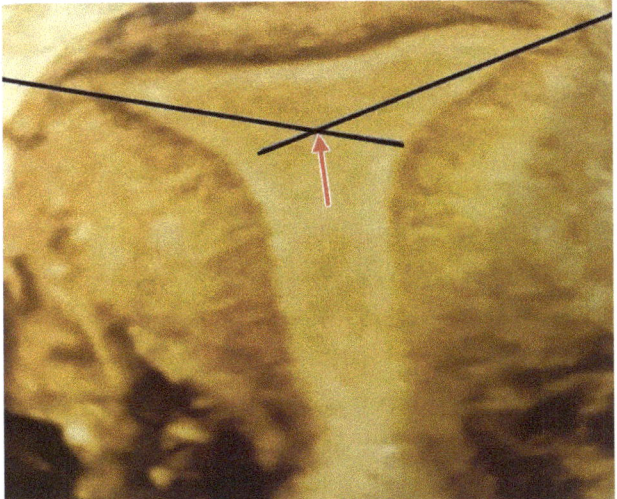

Fig. 4: Intersection of the lines drawn through the uterine cornua, indicating point of maximum implantation.

Catheters

There is a wide variety of embryo transfer catheters available for clinical use. They differ in diameter, length, malleability, presence of an outer sheath, stiffness, material memory, and characteristics of the tip.

The full benefits of soft catheter are better appreciated if an outer sheath is minimally used and stopped just before the internal os, since irritation of the internal os is believed to trigger uterine contractions. The inner soft catheter is better appreciated if it has air bubbles or an echogenic tip, since it is easier to visualize in real-time ultrasound and makes the transfer easier.

Technique

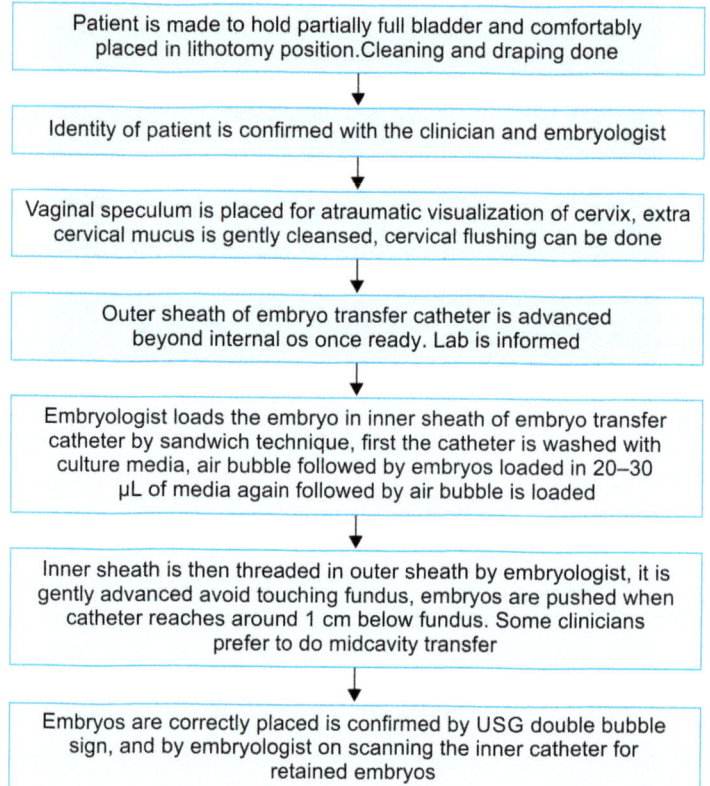

Conclusion

Embryo transfer is the most crucial step in ART. Embryo transfer will determine the success of clinical pregnancy rate. It has to be performed by an experienced clinician. One needs to encompass a tender loving care attitude to get the best results.

CHAPTER 6

Role of Laparoscopy Before IVF

Priya Bhave Chittawar

INTRODUCTION

In vitro fertilization (IVF) was invented as cure for tubal factor infertility and has now expanded its scope for a myriad of factors thus maximizing a couple's chances of conception. Hysteroscopy provides the opportunity to directly visualize the uterine cavity and enable a nuanced evaluation of the same. Laparoscopy enables the surgeon to visualize the uterus, tubes and ovary, and their relationship to each other.

Although routine laparoscopy-hysteroscopy is not recommended in workup of an infertile couple, there are a few scenarios where prior hysteroscopy and laparoscopy or their combination helps in optimization of the IVF outcomes. Recent trials have also confirmed the fact that routine hysteroscopy prior to IVF in unscreened population or a patient with a normal USG finding is not beneficial.

LAPAROSCOPY

Laparoscopic tubal delinking or salpingectomy in patients with communicating hydrosalpinx increases the pregnancy rates by 50% in patients undergoing IVF. Various hypotheses explaining this include mechanical hindrance to implantation, endometrial receptivity, and the emrbyotoxic nature of hydrosalpingeal fluid.

Genital tuberculosis (TB) has a nonspecific manifestations and is quite prevalent in Southeast Asia. The diagnosis is often delayed until fibrotic stages where the tubes have already been damaged beyond repair. Laparohysteroscopy for confirmation of etiology followed by anti-TB treatment (ATT) is beneficial in patients with suspicious history and suspected clinical findings, e.g., mid-tubal block.

Role of laparoscopic surgery in patients with endometriosis is a little tricky. We have to thoroughly discuss the pros and cons of surgery with patient considering their fertility outcomes. Subsets of patients who definitely benefit from laparoscopy include those with advanced endometriosis with severe symptoms and inaccessible ovaries.

HYSTEROSCOPY

Hysteroscopy in patients with suspicious USG findings helps in achieving optimal status of the endometrium essential for implantation.

Removal of polyp is associated with improved pregnancy rates compared to control. Removal of uterine septum is associated with improved obstetrical outcomes, however, recent trials challenge this long-believed notion.

In patients with uterine adhesions, hysteroscopic adhesiolysis and metroplasty are safe and effective approaches to maximize implantation rates.

Subtle findings of hyperemia, stromal edema and micropolyps are useful in diagnosis of patients with chronic endometritis. Treatment for the same is, however not well established with improved pregnancy rates.

CHAPTER 7

Role of Adjuvants in Assisted Reproductive Techniques

Atishay Jain

■ INTRODUCTION

Assisted reproductive techniques (ARTs) have been widely performed for couples suffering from infertility. About one million couples annually conceive with ART around the world. Despite several path-breaking inventions in the field they still have a success rate per cycle of between 19% and 22%, in spite of the advancement in stimulation protocols, quality control in embryology, and various other aspects of ART.[1,2] This low success rate has lead of the development of other add-ons to increase the success rates of in vitro fertilization (IVF) cycles. Adjuvant or add-ons are agents, tools or procedures performed along with the ART–IVF or intracytoplasmic sperm injection (ICSI) to improve the fertility outcomes by increasing the number of oocytes, oocyte or sperm quality or endometrial receptivity. Most of the studies undertaken are still in the initial stages and have not shown clear evidence of improving success rates and to routinely use them for patients.

Most commonly used adjuvant therapies can be broadly classified in the following ways:[3]
1. *Adjuvants for ovarian response/oocyte:*
    - Androgens—dehydroepiandrostenedione (DHEA) and testosterone
    - Growth hormone (GH)
    - Metformin
    - Antioxidants
    - Artificial oocyte activation (AOA)
2. *Adjuvants for sperm:*
    - Sperm DNA fragmentation tests and antioxidants
    - Advanced sperm selection techniques including:
        – Intracytoplasmic morphologically selected sperm injection (IMSI)
        – Physiological intracytoplasmic sperm injection (PICSI)
3. *Adjuvants for embryos:*
    - Time-lapse embryo imaging
    - Embryo glue
    - Assisted hatching (AH)
    - Elective "freeze-all" cycle

- Preimplantation genetic screening (PGS)/preimplantation genetic testing for aneuploidy (PGT-A)
- Autologous endometrial co-culture
4. *Adjuvants for endometrium/implantation:*
   - Estrogen
   - Aspirin
   - Heparin
   - Vasodilators—Nitroglycerine (NTG), Sildenafil, L-arginine.
   - Uterine relaxants—β2-adrenergic antagonists, piroxicam, atosiban
   - Endometrial scratching/endometrial injury (EI)
   - Reproductive immunology testing and potential therapies:
     - Corticosteroids
     - Intravenous immunoglobulin (IVIG)
     - Anti-tumor necrosis factor-α (anti-TNF-α) agents
     - Intralipid infusion
     - Granulocyte colony-stimulating factor (G-CSF)
     - Autologous platelet rich plasma (PRP) therapy
     - Intrauterine hCG administration
     - Autologous peripheral blood mononuclear cells (PBMC)

Most commonly used adjuvants are discussed below.

Androgens

Current evidence highlights the evidence of using androgens in poor responders as moderate.

Dehydroepiandrostenedione is a widely used adjuvant in poor ovarian responders. DHEA is a dietary supplement. It helps to enhance follicular function in older women with diminished follicular reserve by increasing the production of insulin-like growth factor-1 (IGF-1) and augmenting estradiol production in granulosa cells, acting as a precursor of androstenedione and testosterone in the theca cells. In turn leading to improvement in the number of antral follicles available for stimulation.

Testosterone has been used as an adjuvant in poor ovarian responders. It is usually administered transdermally (testosterone gel 12.5 mg once daily for 21 days or 2.5 mg testosterone patch for 5 days prior to ovarian stimulation).

Growth Hormone

It regulates the effect of FSH on the granulosa cells of the ovary by increasing the synthesis of IGF-1 and has a role in improving ovarian function including follicular development, estrogen synthesis, and oocyte maturation.[4] Currently studies have been inconclusive regarding the use of GH and the dosage of this hormone.

Metformin

Women with polycystic ovarian syndrome (PCOS) are more insulin-resistant and hyperinsulinemic than normal women. Metformin helps to decrease the ovarian secretion of vascular endothelial growth factor (VEGF) which helps in the development of ovarian hyperstimulation syndrome (OHSS). Available evidence suggests that metformin may have some beneficial effects in women with PCOS undergoing IVF by reducing the risk of developing OHSS and increasing the pregnancy rates.

Antioxidants

Oxidative stress can lead to cell membrane lipid peroxidation, cellular protein oxidation, and DNA damage, causing a negative effect upon the oocyte, the embryo, and implantation.[5] Antioxidants act as scavengers of oxygen free radicals and prevent this oxidative damage. Various antioxidants have been studied such as acetyl-cysteine, melatonin, L-arginine, myo-inositol, D-chiro-inositol, carnitine, selenium, vitamin E, vitamin B complex, vitamin C, vitamin D + calcium, CoQ10, pentoxifylline, and omega-3-polyunsaturated fatty acids. Current evidence has shown there is limited evidence to prove the role of antioxidants in improving pregnancy rates.

Artificial Oocyte Activation

Scientists have used calcium ionophores to artificially induce oocyte activation at the time of fertilization in an IVF/ICSI cycle. Increases calcium ion concentration around the ooplasm immediately following sperm-oocyte fusion and thereby has been shown to increase fertilization rates.

AOA using calcium ionophores may improve fertilization rates in ICSI cycles, where the oocyte and sperm have failed to activate in previous treatment cycles.

Sperm DNA Fragmentation Tests and Antioxidants

Various tests, such as TUNEL, Comet, SCD assay, SCSA, and 8-OHdG test, are available to test sperm DNA fragmentation but it has been concluded that current methods for assessing sperm DNA integrity do not reliably predict treatment outcomes and cannot be recommended routinely for clinical use.

Advanced Sperm Selection Techniques

IMSI is a sperm selection technique which involves using a microscope to view sperm under very high magnification (over 6000×).

PICSI involves placing sperm with hyaluronic acid and identifying the sperm that can bind to HA and these sperm are selected for use in treatment. Currently there is not enough evidence to support the routine use of advanced sperm selection techniques over standard ICSI.[6]

Assisted Hatching

Many scientists proposed that breach in the zona pellucida may help implantation in some patients.

Chemical or laser-assisted hatching has been proposed to help a hardened zona break and create channels for exchange of metabolites, growth factors, and signals between the embryos and endometrium.

Currently, AH is not recommended because it has not been shown to improve pregnancy rates

Freeze-all Cycle

Few studies stated that pregnancy rates are increased by using frozen embryo transfers (FETs) rather than fresh transfer, but have found inconsistent results for the same.

Preimplantation Genetic Screening

Numerical chromosomal abnormalities of either meiotic or mitotic origin in preimplantation embryos have been regarded as the main reason for implantation failure, miscarriage, and prolonged time to pregnancy in IVF.

Current studies do not provide sufficient evidence to consider PGS/PGT-A as an effective adjuvant therapy to improve pregnancy rates.

Estrogen

Estrogen can be used as an adjuvant for follicular priming and endometrial development in women undergoing IVF cycles, but the available evidence does not recommend routine estradiol supplementation for endometrial development in the luteal phase support of fresh IVF cycles.

Aspirin

Acetylsalicylic acid (Aspirin) is a nonsteroidal anti-inflammatory agent that works by inhibition of cyclooxygenase enzyme in platelets and reduction of prostaglandin synthesis. It causes a shift from thromboxane A_2 to prostacyclin, thereby leading to vasodilation and increased peripheral blood flow including uterine blood flow leading to an increase in endometrial receptivity and implantation rates. Although routine use of aspirin has not been concluded through current evidence.

Heparin

Both unfractionated and low molecular weight heparin (LMWH) have been used to promote successful invasion of trophoblasts in the presence of antiphospholipid syndrome as heparin exerts its antithrombotic effect by inhibition of factor Xa and thrombin.

It has been studied that heparin modulates endometrial receptivity and decidualization of endometrial stromal cells, and improves implantation. However, there is insufficient evidence to provide their effective role.

Vasodilators

Various agents such as nitroglycerine, sildenafil citrate and L-argenine have been studied but there is no sufficient evidence to support their role in improving IVF outcomes.

Uterine Relaxants

In IVF cycles, uterine activity is increased compared with that in natural cycle conception. Adverse uterine activity at the time of embryo transfer can occur due to early timing of transfer in the luteal phase, mechanical stimulation, and supraphysiological hormonal environment. Atosiban, β2-adrenergic antagonists, nitroglycerine and piroxicam have been studied but evidence to support their beneficial role is insufficient.

Endometrial Scratching

Various authors concluded that the role of endometrial scratching does not improve the chance of pregnancy for women undergoing ART.

Corticosteroids

Due to their anti-inflammatory and immune-suppressive activity and hence it has been postulated that it might improve the intrauterine environment by reducing endometrial proinflammatory cytokines production and natural killer (NK) cell activity.

In spite of their function, there is no convincing evidence to prove their beneficial role.

Granulocyte Colony-stimulating Factor

It has been postulated that G-CSF has a direct role in promoting endometrial growth but various studies have proven that there is not sufficient data on its vital role.

Autologous Platelet-rich Plasma

The high concentrations of growth factors, cytokines, and platelets in the concentrate have been the theoretical basis for its application as a regenerative and tissue-healing agent. PRP was administered through ultrasound-guided injection into the ovaries, subsequent improvement was reported in ovarian reserve markers and in ovarian response to gonadotropin stimulation for IVF. Recent studies have shown the positive effects in promoting endometrial and follicular growth and gestation in assisted reproduction cycles.[7-9] But due to lack of large trials, the role has been experimental.

REFERENCES

1. De Geyter C, Calhaz-Jorge C, Kupka MS, Wyns C, Mocanu E, Motrenko T, et al. ART in Europe, 2014: results generated from European registries by ESHRE: The European IVF-monitoring Consortium (EIM) for the European Society of Human Reproduction and Embryology (ESHRE). Hum Reprod. 2018;33:1586-601.
2. Adamson GD, de Mouzon J, Chambers GM, Zegers-Hochschild F, Mansour R, Ishihara O, et al. International Committee for Monitoring Assisted Reproductive Technology: world report on assisted reproductive technology, 2011. Fertil Steril. 2018;110:1067-80.
3. Zemyarska MS. Is it ethical to provide IVF add-ons when there is no evidence of a benefit if the patient requests it? J Med Ethics 2019;45:346-50. doi: 10.1136/medethics-2018-104983.
4. Howles CM, Loumaye E, Germond M, Yates R, Brinsden P, Healy D, et al. Does growth hormone-releasing factor assist follicular development in poor responder patients undergoing ovarian stimulation for in-vitro fertilization? Hum Reprod. 1999;14:1939-43.
5. Ruder EH, Hartman TJ, Blumberg J, Goldman MB. Oxidative stress and antioxidants: exposure and impact on female fertility. Hum Reprod Update. 2008;14:345-57.
6. Harper J, Jackson E, Sermon K, Aitken RJ, Harbottle S, Mocanu E, et al. Adjuncts in the IVF laboratory: where is the evidence for "add-on" interventions? Hum Reprod. 2017;32:485-91. doi: 10.1093/humrep/dex004.
7. Chang Y, Li J, Chen Y, Wei L, Yang X, Shi Y, et al. Autologous platelet rich plasma promotes endometrial growth and improves pregnancy outcome during in vitro fertilization. Int J Clin Exp Med. 2015;8:1286-90.
8. Bos-Mikich A, de oliveira R, Frantz N. Platelet-rich plasma therapy and reproductive medicine. J Assist Reprod Genet. 2018;35:753-6.
9. Kim H, Shin JE, Koo HS, Kwon H, Choi DH, Kim JH. Effect of autologous platelet-rich plasma treatment on refractory thin endometrium during the frozen embryo transfer cycle: a pilot study. Front Endocrinol. 2019;10:61. doi: 10.3389/fendo.2019.00061.

CHAPTER 8

Ovarian Reserve Markers

Sunita Arora

■ INTRODUCTION

Ovarian reserve testing at any point of time determines the fertility potential of a woman. As clearly evident woman in later stages of life when menstrual cycle becomes irregular, have lower ovarian reserve as compared woman in reproductive years.[1] Studies indicate that there can be significant difference in ovarian reserve of women of same age group also.[2]

Tests for ovarian reserve include blood tests to measure hormone levels as well as ultrasound imaging of the ovaries. Biochemical tests are follicle-stimulating hormone (FSH), estradiol (E2), inhibin B to be measured on day 2-5 of menses and anti-Müllerian hormone (AMH) which is independent of the day of the cycle.

FSH measured on day 2 or 3 is the most widely used test to assess ovarian response to stimulation.[3] It has intercycle and intracycle variation, that limits the reliability of a single measurement.[4,5] Since ovarian ageing begins several years before any elevation of FSH levels, a normal level cannot rule out poor ovarian response. FSH can predict a poor response only at very high levels, so will be helpful to a limited population as a screening test for poor response,[6,7] thus should be combined with other markers for counseling purpose.

Estradiol levels vary in the same cycle, peak in late follicular and mid-luteal phase. This should also be combined with FSH levels to assess diminished reserve. Elevated E2 levels (>60-80 pg/mL) may also lead to an artificially normal FSH, where higher E2 levels lead to feedback suppression of FSH. Conversely, E2 levels < 20 pg/mL on day 3 can mean normal ovarian function, hypogonadotropic hypogonadism (HH), or ovarian failure. So, an elevated day 3, E2 can mean diminished ovarian reserve. Hence, E2 levels always needed to be interpreted with great caution.

Serum concentrations of AMH, produced by granulosa cells of early follicles, are gonadotropin independent and, therefore, remain relatively consistent within and between menstrual cycles in both normal, young, ovulating women and women with infertility.[8-11] The number of the small antral follicles is related to the size of the primordial follicle pool. As age advances antral follicles decrease and AMH production appears to diminish and become undetectable at and after menopause.[12] AMH levels strongly correlate with basal antral follicle count (AFC) measured by transvaginal ultrasonography.[13] Unlike other biochemical markers, it can be measured on any day of the cycle[10,11] and does not exhibit intercycle variability.[8] Various threshold values, 0.2–1.26 ng/mL, have been used to identify poor responders with 80–87% sensitivity and 64–93% specificity.[14-16]

AMH is a more sensitive measure of ovarian reserve than FSH and tends to decline before FSH rises. Basal FSH and E2 levels may provide added information in women with very low AMH.

Inhibin B is a glycoprotein secreted by preantral follicles, and a direct measure of the follicular pool. Levels start declining with age and falls 4 years prior to menopause. As the level of inhibin B declines it lowers the central negative feedback leading to high FSH levels in late luteal and early follicular phase.

AFC is the number, antral follicles in both ovaries combined together, as observed on transvaginal sonography on day 2 or 3 of cycle. Most studies describe antral follicles as those measuring between 2 and 10 mm in greatest two dimensions across the ovary. Repeated measurements have shown that there is only a limited intercycle variability.[17] A count of 8–10 in each ovary is considered a predictor of normal response. AFC is considered one of the best markers for ovarian response as compared to total ovarian volume, and blood levels of FSH, E2, and inhibin B on day 3 of cycle but it lacks sensitivity and specificity to predict the pregnancy outcome.[18,19]

Ovarian reserve tests have a moderate ability to predict poor or hyper ovarian response, and are useful in choosing the type of treatment protocol for ovarian stimulation. These tests should not be used to exclude any woman from in vitro fertilization (IVF) treatment. Evidence shows that AFC and AMH appear to be the most useful markers of ovarian reserve, and age being an important indicator. This might help women make enhanced fertility choices in cases of delayed child-bearing and timely egg preservation.

REFERENCES

1. Hansen KR, Craig LB, Zavy MT, Klein NA, Soules MR. Ovarian primordial and non-growing follicle counts according to the Stages of Reproductive Aging Workshop (STRAW) staging system. Menopause. 2012;19:164-71.
2. Hansen KR, Knowlton NS, Thyer AC, Charleston JS, Soules MR, Klein NA. A new model of reproductive aging: the decline in ovarian nongrowing follicle number from birth to menopause. Hum Reprod. 2008;23:699-708.
3. Scott RT, Toner JP, Muasher SJ, Oehninger S, Robinson S, Rosenwaks Z. Follicle-stimulating hormone levels on cycle day 3 are predictive of in vitro fertilization outcome. Fertil Steril. 1989;51:651-4.
4. Scott RT Jr, Hofmann, GE, Oehninger S, Muasher SJ. Intercycle variability of day 3 follicle-stimulating hormone levels and its effect on stimulation quality in in vitro fertilization. Fertil Steril. 1990;54:297-302.
5. Kwee J, Schats R, McDonnell J, Lambalk CB, Schoemaker J. Intercycle variability of ovarian reserve tests: results of a prospective randomized study. Hum Reprod. 2004;19:590-5.

6. Bancsi LF, Broekmans FJ, Mol BW, Habbema JD, teVelde ER. Performance of basal follicle-stimulating hormone in the prediction of poor ovarian response and failure to become pregnant after in vitro fertilization: a meta-analysis. Fertil Steril. 2003;79:1091-100.
7. Broekmans FJ, Kwee J, Hendriks DJ, Mol BW, Lambalk CB. A systematic review of tests predicting ovarian reserve and IVF outcome. Hum Reprod Update. 2006;12:685-718.
8. Fanchin R, Taieb J, Lozano DH, Ducot B, Frydman R, Bouyer J. High reproducibility of serum anti-Müllerian hormone measurements suggests a multi-staged follicular secretion and strengthens its role in the assessment of ovarian follicular status. Hum Reprod. 2005;20:923-7.
9. Tsepelidis S, Devreker F, Demeestere I, Flahaut A, Gervy C, Englert Y. Stable serum levels of anti-Müllerian hormone during the menstrual cycle: a prospective study in normo-ovulatory women. Hum Reprod. 2007;22:1837-40.
10. La Marca A, Stabile G, Artensio AC, Volpe A. Serum anti-Müllerian hormone throughout the human menstrual cycle. Hum Reprod. 2006;21:3103-7.
11. Hehenkamp WJ, Looman CW, Themmen AP, de Jong FH, teVelde ER, Broekmans FJ. Anti-Müllerian hormone levels in the spontaneous menstrual do not show substantial fluctuation. J Clin Endocrinol Metab. 2006; 91:4057-63.
12. de Vet A, Laven JS, de Jong FH, Themmen AP, Fauser BC. Anti-Müllerian hormone serum levels: aputative marker for ovarian aging. Fertil Steril. 2002;77:357-62.
13. Broer SL, Dólleman M, Opmeer BC, Fauser BC, Mol BW, Broekmans FJ. AMH and AFC as predictors of excessive response in controlled ovarian hyperstimulation: a meta-analysis. Hum Reprod Update. 2011;17:46-54.
14. Muttukrishna S, McGarrigle H, Wakim R, Khadum I, Ranieri DM, Serhal P. Antral follicle count, anti-Müllerian hormone and inhibin B: predictors of ovarian response in assisted reproductive technology? BJOG. 2005;112:1384-90.
15. Tremellen KP, Kolo M, Gilmore A, Lekamge DN. Anti-Müllerian hormone as a marker of ovarian reserve. Aust N Z J Obstet Gynaecol. 2005;45:20-4.
16. La Marca A, Giulini S, Tirelli A, Bertucci E, Marsella T, Xella S, et al. Anti-Müllerian hormone measurement on any day of the menstrual cycle strongly predicts ovarian response in assisted reproductive technology. Hum Reprod. 2007;22:766-71.
17. Bancsi LF, Broekmans FJ, Looman CW, Habbema JD, teVelde ER. Impact of repeated antral follicle counts on the prediction of poor ovarian response in women undergoing in vitro fertilization. Fertil Steril. 2004;81:35-41.
18. Maheshwari A, Fowler P, Bhattacharya S. Assessment of ovarian reserve—should we perform tests of ovarian reserve routinely? Hum Reprod. 2006;21:2729-35.
19. Hendriks DJ, Kwee J, Mol BW, Te Velde ER, Broekmans FJ. Ultrasonography as a tool for the prediction of outcome in IVF patients: a comparative meta-analysis of ovarian volume and antral follicle count. Fertil Steril. 2007;87:764-75.

CHAPTER 9

Premature Ovarian Ageing, Role of Platelet Rich Plasma and Stem Cells

Niket Patel

ABSTRACT

Premature ovarian ageing (POA) is a grave condition that affects women leading to infertility due to lack of available oocytes for fertilization. Egg or oocyte donation remains an option for these patients.

Stem cell research and regenerative medicine have became integral in the field of obstetrics and gynecology. With the explosion of technologies, there is a critical need to understand properties and to expand the uses of stem cells and platelet rich plasma (PRP) directed at treatments for infertility. Notably, there is great interest in regeneration of aged or damaged tissues by stem cell-based and PRP-based technologies. To date, there are no stem cell-based therapies available to the larger public outside of clinical trials. Specifically, there are no proven stem cell based means to improve reproductive function. However, a promising avenue of research includes the development of therapies from adult stem cells of limited potency in the treatment of reproductive tract alterations, such as erectile dysfunction or damaged endometrial lining. Upon the activation of platelets, the alpha granules release several biologically active factors, including platelet-derived growth factor (PDGF), transforming growth factor beta (TGF-β), insulin-like growth factor-1 (IGF-1), vascular endothelial growth factor (VEGF), epidermal growth factor (EGF), basic fibroblast growth factor (bFGF), and proinflammatory cytokines. Results of many studies indicate that regenerative medicine has the potential to restore fertility with use of stem cells and PRP. The treatment was found to be effective in ovarian rejuvenation, increasing endometrial thickness, development of embryo in vitro, in better implantation of embryo in patient with repeated implantation failure (RIF), increasing the motility of sperm, reversing the damage to the testis, etc., and has potential to generate functional gametes. Moreover, our own experience at Akanksha Hospital and Research Institute, Gujarat, India, of 4 Years in the same field has exposed us to many new advances.

CONCLUSION

Development in the field of regenerative medicine and its clinical applications will provide effective treatment options in patients with various conditions lead to infertility. So, more clinical trials with use of regenerative medicine should be encouraged, as it seems to have the potential to be a future regimen for infertility.

Newer Stimulation Protocols: PPOS and DuoStim

Manjiri Valsangkar

INTRODUCTION

It has been observed in last decade that there has been a 10% rise in the incidence of diminished ovarian reserve in young infertility patients. It poses as a major limiting factor for in vitro fertilization (IVF) success due to reduction in quality and quantity of oocytes. Accurate diagnostic evaluation and individualized controlled ovarian stimulation (COS) is the key to success. Traditionally, the long agonist protocol has been the mainstay of treatment in DOR patients, however, it is expensive, dose of gonadotropins and duration of treatment is very long.

Researchers have worked in this direction to limit duration and cost of treatment, and newer stimulation protocols have been tried and various randomized controlled trials (RCTs) published in this regard.

PROGESTIN-PRIMED OVARIAN STIMULATION (PPOS) PROTOCOL (FIG. 1)

Kuang and colleagues conducted a primary randomized study on PPOS. They added medroxyprogesterone acetate 10 mg BD daily to gonadotropin-induced

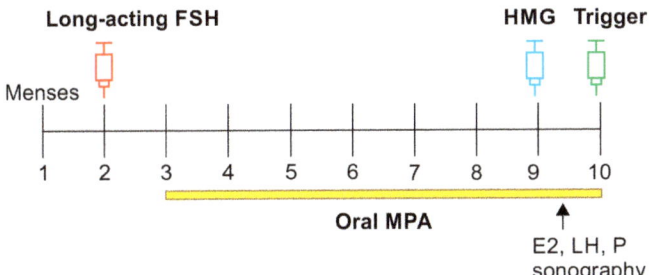

Fig. 1: PPOS protocol.
(E2: estradiol; FSH: follicle-stimulating hormone; hMG: human menopausal gonadotropin; MPA: medroxyprogesterone acetate; P: progesterone)
Source: Yu S, Long H, Chang HY, Liu Y, Gao H, Zhu J, et al. New application of dydrogesterone as a part of a progestin-primed ovarian stimulation protocol for IVF: a randomized controlled trial including 516 first IVF/ICSI cycles. Hum Reprod. 2018;33:229-37.

stimulation in the follicular phase along with low dose gonadotropins till the day of trigger. This study showed comparative pregnancy, implantation and miscarriage rates as compared to conventional protocols. This protocol effectively stops the premature estrogen-induced LH surge and gives comparative results.

Nanako Iwami and co-workers compared the rates of ongoing and clinical pregnancies between the antagonist regimen and the PPOS protocol. They used oral dydrogesterone (OD) 20 mg/day and human menopausal gonadotropin (hMG) in the PPOS protocol. They concluded that the rates of ongoing and clinical pregnancies were similar in both groups. Additionally, they also included normal responders in addition to hyper-responders such as polycystic ovary syndrome (PCOS). In a pilot study, a short protocol was compared with the PPOS protocol in PCOS patients. This article reported no significant differences in the number of collected oocyte and the incidence of ongoing pregnancy.

DUAL OVARIAN STIMULATION (DUOSTIM) PROTOCOL (FIG. 2)

Recent evidence suggests that follicular development occurs in a wave-like pattern at least 2 or 3 cohorts of follicles recruitable in one menstrual cycle. This is different from previous understanding that follicles can be recruited only during the follicular phase. This novel concept gave rise to DuoStim for diminished ovarian reserve patients with a limited cohort of follicles. DuoStim strategy (double stimulation in the follicular and luteal phase of the same ovarian cycle) in patients who are poor ovarian responders also called Shanghai protocol. In order to participate, patients

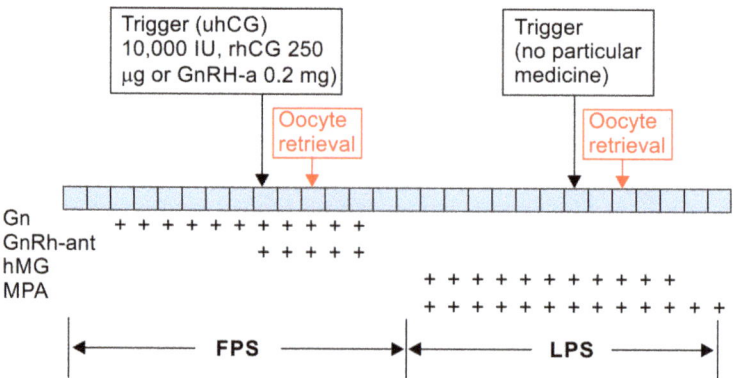

Fig. 2: Steps of ovarian stimulation with DuoStim protocol.
(uhCG: urinary human chorionic gonadotropin; rhCG: recombinant hCG; MPA: medroxyprogesterone acetate; GnRH-a: gonadotropin-releasing hormone agonist; GnRH-ant: GnRH antagonists; hMG: human menopausal gonadotropin; FPS: follicular phase stimulation; LPS: luteal phase stimulation)

had to meet at least two of the following criteria: age over 40 years; a history of ovarian surgery; previous treatment using conventional protocols that yielded less than three oocytes; antral follicle count of less than 5 on menstrual cycle day 2–3; and basal serum follicle-stimulating hormone (FSH) concentration between 10 and 19 IU/L. Follicular phase recruitment was done with letrozole along with 225 IU hMG or recombinant FSH (rFSH) followed by trigger with gonadotropin-releasing hormone agonist (GnRH-a) in primary cycle, vitrification of all embryos, accumulation and subsequent transfer in next cycle. After the ovum pick-up, second stimulation was immediately started with hMG and trigger with agonist or hCG in luteal phase cycle followed by vitrification of embryos. It was concluded that luteal phase embryos gave comparable results as conventional protocols.

CHAPTER 11

Vitrification: The Game-changer

Parasuram Gopinath

INTRODUCTION

There have been several landmark events in the evolution of assisted reproductive technology (ART) procedures and one such event was the introduction of *vitrification*. For a very long time the surplus embryos produced during your routine ART treatment had to be discarded and if the treatment becomes unsuccessful, the patient has to undergo the whole treatment once again. This challenge was leading to significant rise in cost, and inconvenience to the patients and hence the introduction of cryopreservation of surplus embryos came into existence. The initial method of cryopreservation was slow freezing with its biggest challenge being suboptimal post-thaw survival and the dependence on equipment. This is when the process of vitrification or ultra-fast cooling of embryos was introduced, which was indeed a game-changer in the field of infertility with its high post-thaw survival and convenience of procedure. The current evidence is quite clear that vitrification is now the preferred technique of cryopreservation in most of the in vitro fertilization (IVF) centers around the world.

Vitrification is the rapid cooling of liquid medium in the absence of ice crystal formation. The solution forms an amorphous glass as a result of rapid cooling by direct immersion of the embryos in a polyethylene (PE) straw into liquid nitrogen. It is considered as an ideal way of storing embryos and oocytes for future use. With the increased confidence in vitrification, the whole trend in ART process is moving to a freeze-all strategy to improve outcomes. With the introduction of procedures such as preimplantation genetic testing of embryos, role of vitrification has become more relevant.

There have been several aspects in vitrification that has been of concern like the possible effect of the procedure per se or the toxicity of the cryoprotectant solution. Even though there is an increased incidence of large for gestational babies after frozen embryo transfer (FET) and there are no other adverse fetal or neonatal outcomes reported in pregnancies from frozen embryos compared to fresh embryos. Irrespective of the type of gamete (oocyte especially) or stage of embryo whether it is day 3 or day 4 embryos or blastocyst or even if it has been biopsied, vitrification is still considered the preferred method of cryopreservation.

The biggest challenge with regards to cryopreservation is that the procedure is skill dependent and hence the variability in its performance across various clinics. Hence it is important to train your staff and customize the procedure as per your lab for optimal outcome.

CHAPTER 12

Artificial Intelligence in IVF: A Need

Sayali Kandari, Keshav Malhotra

INTRODUCTION

The birth of the first in vitro fertilization (IVF) baby in 1978 was a remarkable milestone in the field of human reproductive biology. In the last 40 years, the clinical practice and embryology laboratory has advanced from bell jars to artificial intelligence (AI) driven time-lapse incubators.

THE PROGRESS OF ASSISTED REPRODUCTIVE TECHNOLOGY (ART)

Improved culture media and culture systems, the expanding horizons of IVF including new advances in intracytoplasmic sperm injection (ICSI), vitrification, morphokinetics and lab QA/QC have increased the number of measurable parameters from single digits to thousands of data points with more than 300 key performance indicators and counting (Alpha, ESHRE good practice guidelines). So the question arises: Is human intervention enough?

WHAT IS ARTIFICIAL INTELLIGENCE?

Artificial intelligence can be classified into three different types of systems: *analytical, human-inspired,* and *humanized artificial intelligence*. We deal only with analytical AI in the field of reproductive medicine. The prime goal is to allow data collation and real-time analysis of millions of data points. The components of AI application are: *Risk stratification; threshold modeling, machine learning (ML), training phase, algorithm development, prediction analysis, gold standard validation, next version RS and TM (Point 1)*. The most recent example is the use of AI to evaluate risk in recurrent miscarriage at ESHRE Annual Meeting 2019, Vienna.

CAN ARTIFICIAL INTELLIGENCE ADVANCE ART?

Reproductive experts can determine the best treatment for the individual infertility of patients by incorporating AI and ML models (Siristatidis et al., 2016). Infertility patients can be provided with the most appropriate therapy, increasing the successful pregnancy rates and reducing the financial burden. At the social level, unnecessary use of medical resources can be avoided leading to a reduction of healthcare costs (Senders et al., 2018).

Up to two-thirds of patients experience failed cycles, but the hope is now that AI systems might be able to flag the most viable embryos. A very recent study from Australia concluded that the agreement between embryologists selecting a single day 5 embryo for transfer was generally good, although not optimal, even among experienced embryologists (Storr A et al., interobserver and intraobserver agreement between embryologists during the selection of a single day 5 embryo for transfer: a multicenter study).

Sixteen AI and ML approaches were reported at 2018 annual congresses of the American Society for Reproductive Biology (ASRM) and the European Society for Human Reproduction and Embryology (ESHRE). Nearly every aspect of patient care was investigated, including sperm morphology, sperm identification, identification of empty or oocyte-containing follicles, predicting embryo cell stages, predicting blastocyst formation from oocytes, assessing human blastocyst quality, predicting live birth from blastocysts, improving embryo selection, and for developing optimal IVF stimulation protocols.

Currently, there are three major categories of AI methods widely used in medical applications: ML, natural language processing (NLP), and robotic surgery. The ML method attempts to cluster the features of patients and predict the outcome of diseases by analyzing structured data such as medical imaging and genetic data (Darcy et al., 2016). The NLP method extracts and processes meaningful information from unstructured clinical data, such as electronic medical records (EMRs), to complement the structured data (Nadkarni et al., 2011, Mehta, Devarakonda, 2018). NLP converts the raw data into structured data that the machine can read and few AI solutions available are:

1. ***Eeva test***, which uses time-lapse imaging microscopy to collect data over the length of the embryo's culture period, and an algorithm to predict which embryo has the best chance of progressing.
2. ***IVY***, in Australia, Aengus Tran and his colleagues have developed an AI that 93% of the time correctly predicts particular embryo progress to the fetal heartbeat. The fully automated system analyzes time-lapse video sequences and requires no human input, and thus is not subject to embryologist variability.
3. ***Stork*** developed by Weill Cornell. USA is not commercially available moreover, current data used INCEPTION IV platform for AI development again, using time-lapse images.
4. ***Future fertility*** is working on developing AI for oocyte quality monitoring, focusing on static and time-lapse 2D imaging. They have plans to integrate ultrasound imaging and embryo scoring in their algorithm.

A true AI system uses "deep learning" to refine itself on the fly based on new information. The "learning" in deep learning is achieved through training: hundreds or thousands of data points are fed into the model so that

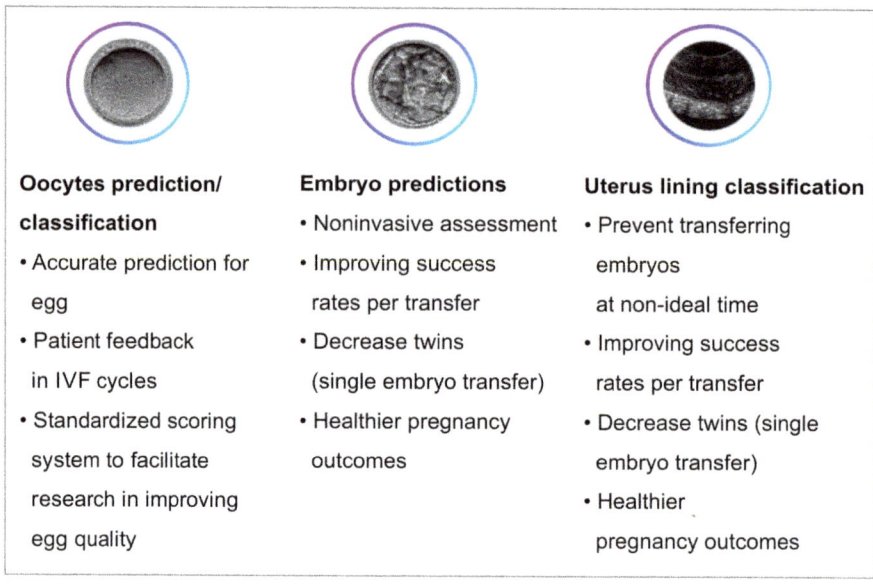

Source: Futurefertility.com.

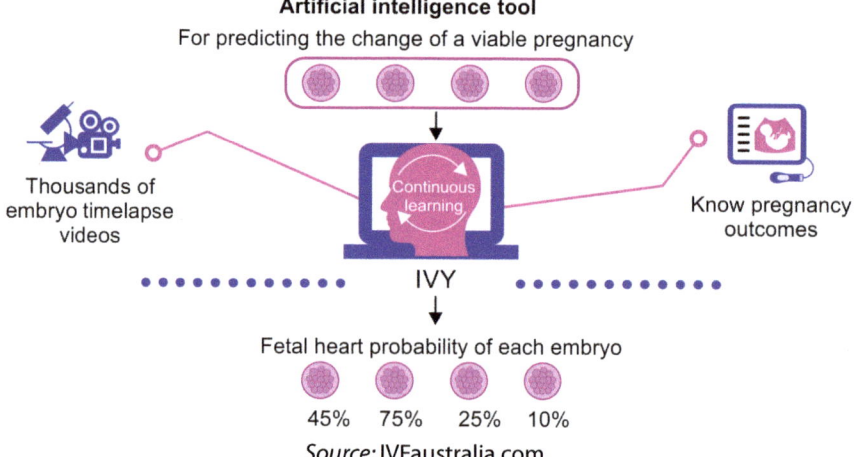

Source: IVFaustralia.com.

future outcomes can be predicted—and then the predictions are compared against actual outcomes.

AI systems for IVF are still in the experimental phase, but the results so far have been promising. Overall, the AI system will be having a high percentage of accuracy, catching small details that signaled poor quality embryos human evaluators could not see. AI can be a useful prescreening

Flowchart 1: Where artificial intelligence can intervene?

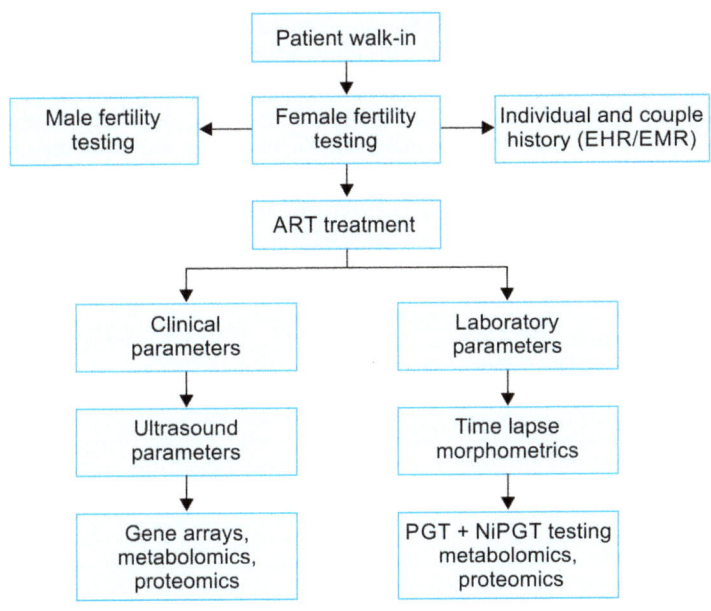

(PGT: preimplantation genetic testing; NiPGT: noninvasive PGT; ART: assisted reproductive technology; EMR: electronic medical record; EHR: electronic health record)
Source: Created by Dr Sayali Kandari for ISAR Newsletter AI in IVF; 2019.

tool that would allow us to identify and genetically test only those embryos which are viable, with a low likelihood of genetic defects. This can result in significant cost savings for patients, and also has the potential to improve pregnancy success. A true "end-to-end" AI for infertility care will have to integrate complex (and diverse) datasets that are currently managed in multiple, incompatible systems—patient demographics and medical histories; drug-treatment regimens, pre-implantation genetic screening; and clinical pregnancy outcome data. It would help embryologists and fertility doctors to choose among several treatment options that have the highest success rates, and accept new information based on the patient's responses to treatments.

In clinical embryology, we do not yet know the feature or set of features that are most predictive of IVF success. It is possible that the most important variable for a successful IVF cycle could still be unknown to science but that could in principle be uncovered by an AI system.

AI technologies have tremendous potential to help the field of infertility medicine to transcend its current narrow focus on individual embryos and uncover new patterns hidden in the patient data for the treatment of stubborn infertility.

FURTHER READING

1. Dimitriadis I, Thirumalaraju P, Kanakasabapathy MJ, et al. Artificial intelligence-enabled system for embryo classification and selection based on image analysis. Fertil Steril. 2019;111:e21.
2. Hardy T, Feng J, Lawrence D, Fullston T, Scott H. Application of artificial intelligence to analysis of the embryonic genome for preimplantation genetic diagnosis. Pathology. 2019;51:S65.
3. Rocha JC, Passalia FJ, Matos FD, et al. A method based on artificial intelligence to fully automatize the evaluation of Bovine blastocyst images. Sci Rep. 2017;7:1-10.
4. Siristatidis C, Pouliakis A, Chrelias C, Kassanos D. Artificial intelligence in IVF: a need. Syst Biol Reprod Med. 2011;57:179-85.
5. Tran A, Cooke S, Illingworth PJ, Gardner DK. Artificial intelligence as a novel approach for embryo selection. Fertil Steril. 2018;110:e430.
6. Wang R, Pan W, Jin L, et al. Artificial intelligence in reproductive medicine. Reproduction. 2019;158:139-54.

CHAPTER 13

Fertility in Women Beyond 35 Years

Mangla Kawade

INTRODUCTION

Age is the single biggest factor affecting a woman's chance to conceive and have a healthy baby. A woman's fertility starts to reduce in her early 30s and more so after the age of 35.

Female infertility is a global medical and social condition caused by various pathophysiological alterations. In a remarkable number of cases, the pathogenesis is not clearly defined, determining indecision concerning the most appropriate treatment choices.

While in developing countries, this condition is related to preventive, diagnostic and therapeutic inadequacy, multiple ovarian endocrine dysfunctions in industrialized nations are apparently associated with improper lifestyles.

Beyond age, a number of lifestyle-related factors, such as excess body weight, obesity, smoking, intense sporting activity, alcohol consumption, drug addiction or abuse of other substances, have adverse influence on female fertility.

Diminished fertility and poor ovarian response pose a conundrum to the experts in the field of reproductive medicine. There is limited knowledge about the risk factors of diminished ovarian reserve other than the iatrogenic ones. One of the leading causes of infertility in women today is *diminished ovarian*

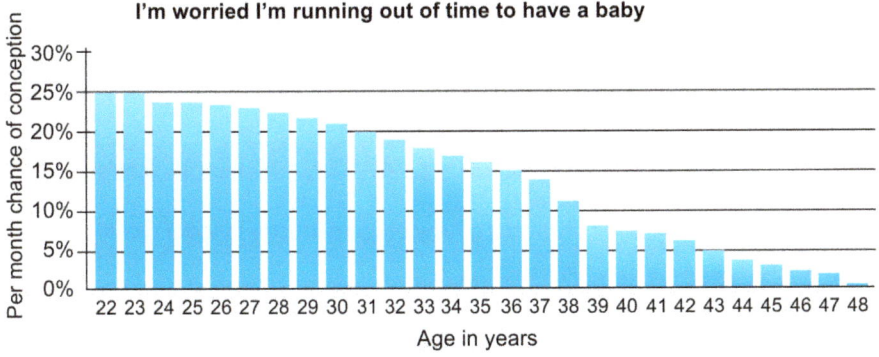

reserve (DOR). DOR is characterized by a low number of eggs in a woman's ovaries and/or with poor quality of the remaining eggs, which boils down to impaired development of the existing eggs, even with assisted reproductive techniques (ARTs). A good number of such women with low ovarian reserve may conceive with their own eggs, if they are given individualized treatment that is tailored for their profile. Such patients should be counseled appropriately for an aggressive approach towards achieving fertility. The sooner the treatment is started, the better the chances of pregnancy.

Ovarian reserve estimation that are used as of now are biochemical, provocative and sonographic imaging of ovaries. The tests used for assessing ovarian reserve include basal day 3 *follicle-stimulating hormone (FSH, introduced in 1998), antral follicle count (AFC, 1997) and anti-Müllerian hormone (AMH, 2002.)* Leader B, et al. studied 5,354 women to examine discordance between AMH and FSH results and found 1 in 5 women with discordant AMH and FSH values defined as AMH < 0.8 ng/mL (concerning) with FSH < 10 IU 0 L (reassuring) or AMH > 0.8 ng/mL (reassuring) with FSH ≥ 10 IU/L (concerning). AMH is more sensitive than FSH in diagnosing DOR, as was found in the study. When ovarian reserve tests are discordant, it's safe to go with an intermediate value between the two and administer an intermediate dose of gonadotropins stimulation.

Age-related abnormal vascularization, oxidative stress, free radical imbalance, toxic and genetic changes, all contribute to the declining oocyte quality, which translates into abnormal fertilization, and disordered embryo implantation.

Poor ovarian response (POR) implies a subnormal follicular response, which means less number of eggs retrieved after ovarian stimulation during in vitro fertilization (IVF). ESHRE defined POR using *Bologna criteria* in order to standardize the definition, since the variability in the definition of POR was striking **(Box 1)**.

POSEIDON's stratification of low prognosis patients in ART: The WHY, the WHAT, and the HOW". "Low prognosis" relates with reduced oocyte number, which can be associated with low or sometimes a normal ovarian reserve and is aggravated by advanced female age. These aspects will ultimately affect

---

Box 1: Bologna criteria for poor responders (ESHRE, 2011).

AT least two of the following criteria:
- Advanced maternal age (≥40 years) or "any other risk factor for poor ovarian response"
- Poor prior response to stimulation (≤3 oocytes when receving at least 150 IU gonadotropin)
- Abnormal ovarian reserve testing (AFC < 7, AMH < 1.1 ng/mL)

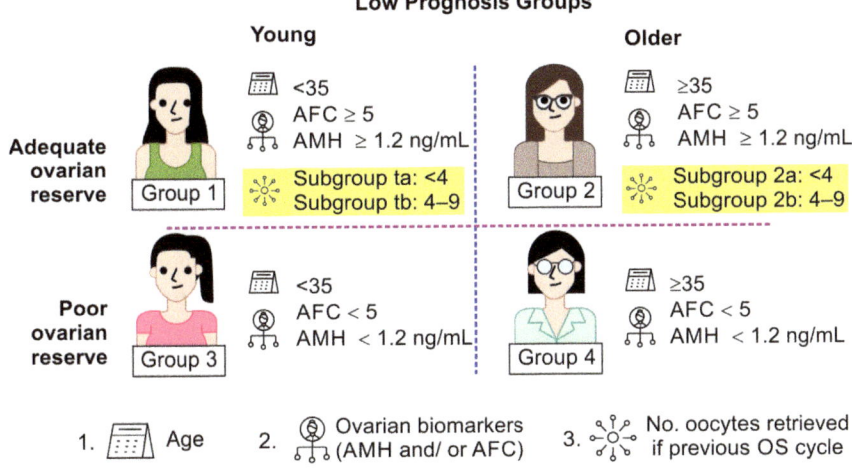

POSEIDON criteria for low prognosis groups.
Source: Esteves SC, Alviggi C, Humaidan P, Fischer R, Andersen CY, Conforti A, et al. The POSEIDON criteria and its measure of success through the eyes of clinicians and embryologists. Front Endocrinol (Lausanne). 2019;10:814.

the number of embryos generated and consequently, the cumulative live birth rate. The novel system relies on female age, ovarian reserve markers, ovarian sensitivity to exogenous gonadotropin, and the number of oocytes retrieved, which will both identify the patients with low prognosis and stratify such patients into one of four groups of women with "expected" or "unexpected" impaired ovarian response to exogenous gonadotropin stimulation.

MANAGEMENT OF PATIENTS BEYOND 35 YEARS

It includes weight reduction if obese, stress, and lifestyle. Adequate intake of antioxidants also supports female reproductive functions since the dietary supplements containing folic acid, β-carotene, vitamin C and E, and an adequate nutritional support of the 1-CC are definitely efficient in shortening the time to conception.

Use of adjuvants [dehydroepiandrosterone (DHEA)], estradiol priming in the luteal phase, recombinant luteinizing hormone (LH), growth hormone (GH), co-treatment use of adjuncts such as androgens, GH, melatonin, aspirin, low molecular weight heparin (LMWH).

Various treatment regimens have been designed to manage the patients with diminished ovarian reserve which include high doses of gonadotropin, natural and modified natural cycles, estrogen priming, supplementation with LH, luteal antagonists and letrozole, oocyte accumulation, dual stimulation/double stimulation (follicular and luteal phase), oocyte donation.

FURTHER READING

1. Broekmans FJ, Kwee J, Hendricks DJ, Mol BW, Lambalk CBA. Systematic review of tests predicting ovarian reserve and IVF outcome. Hum Reprod Update. 2006;12:685-718. doi: 10.1093/humupd/dml034.
2. Cooper AR, Baker VL, Sterling EW, et al. The time is now for a new approach to primary ovarian insufficiency. Fertil Steril. 2012;95:1890-7. doi: 10.1016/j.fertnstert.2010.01.016.
3. Ferraretti AP, Marca L, Fauser BC, Tarlatzis B, Wargund G, et al. ESHRE consensus on the definition of 'poor response' to ovarian stimulation for in vitro fertilization: the Bologna Criteria. Hum Reprod. 2011;26:1616-24. doi: 10.1093/humrep/der092.
4. Gleicher N, Weghofer A, Barad DH. AMH defines, independent of age, low versus good live-birth chances in women with severely diminished ovarian reserve. Fertil Steril. 2010;94:2824-7. doi: 10.1016/j.fertnstert.2010.04.067.
5. Kelsey TW, Anderson RA, Wright P, et al. Data-driven assessment of the human ovarian reserve. Mol Hum Reprod. 2012;18:79-87. doi: 10.1093/molehr/gar059.
6. Kwee J, Schats R, McDowell's J, Lambalk CB, Schoemaker J. Intercycle variability of ovarian reserve tests: results of a prospective randomized study. Hum Reprod. 2004;19:590-5. doi: 10.1093/humrep/deh119.
7. Kyrou D, Kolibeanakis EM, Vanetis EG, Papanekolaon G, et al. How to improve the probability of pregnancy in poor responders undergoing IVF: a systematic review and meta-analysis. Fertil Steril. 2009;91(3):749-66. doi: 10.1016/j.fertnstert.2007.12.077.
8. La Marca A, Sighinolfi G, Raeli D, et al. Anti-Müllerian hormone (AMH) as a predictor marker in assisted reproductive technology (ART). Hum Reprod Update. 2010;16:113-30. doi: 10.1093/humupd/dmp036.
9. Lazer T, Dar S, Shlush E, Al Kudmani BS, Quach K, et al. Comparison of IVF outcomes between minimal stimulation and high-dose stimulation for patients with poor ovarian reserve. Int J Reprod Med. 2014;2014:581451. doi: 10.1155/2014/581451.
10. Nagels HE, Reshworth JR, Serestatides CS, Kroon B. Androgens (DHEA or T) for women undergoing assisted reproduction. Cochrane Database Systematic Review. 2015;(11):CD009749.
11. Rasool S, Shah D. Fertility with early reduction of ovarian reserve: the last straw that breaks the Camel's back. Fertil Res Pract. 2017;3:15. doi: 10.1186/s40738-017-0041-1.
12. Toner JP, Seifee DB. Why we may abandon basal FSH testing: a sea change in determining ovarian reserve using AMH. Fertil Steril. 2013;99:1825-30. doi: 10.1016/j.fertnstert.2013.03.001.

CHAPTER 14

Salient Points of ART Bill, 2020

Shweta Kaul Jha

■ INTRODUCTION

As we know the new Assisted Reproductive Technology (ART) Bill, 2020 has set all the parties involved with ART into a panic mode, this article outlines few take-home points for everyone who is practicing or intends to practice in vitro fertilization (IVF) at India.[1]

■ WHAT ARE PROCEDURES FOR REGISTRATION?

1. No person shall establish any clinic or bank for undertaking ART or to render ART procedures in any form unless such clinic or bank is duly registered under this Act.
2. Every application for registration shall be made to the National Registry through State Board in such form, manner and shall be accompanied by such fees as may be prescribed.
3. Every clinic or bank which is conducting ART, partly or exclusively shall, within a period of 60 days from the date of establishment of the National Registry, apply for registration: Provided that such clinics and banks shall cease to conduct any such counseling or procedures on the expiry of 6 months from the date of commencement of this Act, unless such clinics and banks have applied for registration and is so registered separately or till such application is disposed of, whichever is earlier.
4. No clinics or banks shall be registered under this Act, unless the authority is satisfied that such clinics and banks are in a position to provide such facilities and maintain such equipment and standards including specialized manpower, physical infrastructure and diagnostic facilities as may be prescribed.

Any change in age of couple seeking fertility treatment.
Yes! A welcome positive change.

The clinics shall apply the ART services:
1. To a woman above the legal age of marriage and below the age of 50 years;
2. To a man above the legal age of marriage and below the age of 55 years.

FEW TAKE-HOME POINTS

- Insurance coverage of such amount and for such period as may be prescribed in favor of the oocyte donor by the commissioning couple or woman from an insurance company or an agent recognized by the Insurance Regulatory and Development Authority established under the provisions of the Insurance Regulatory and Development Authority Act, 1999.
- Woman shall not be treated with gametes or embryos derived from more than one man or woman during any one treatment cycle.
- A clinic shall never mix semen from two individuals for the procedures specified under this Act.
- The embryos shall not be split and used for twinning to increase the number of available embryos.
- The collection of gametes posthumously shall be done only if prior consent of the commissioning couple is available.
- Preimplantation genetic testing shall be used to screen the human embryo for known, pre-existing, heritable or genetic diseases or for such other purposes as may be prescribed.
- Donors to be accepted only through ART banks.
- The screening of gamete donors, the collection, screening and storage of semen; and provision of oocyte donor, shall be done only by a bank registered as an independent entity under the provision.
- The banks shall obtain:
  a. Semen from males between 21 and 55 years of age, both inclusive;
  b. Oocytes from females between 23 and 35 years of age; and
  c. Examine the donors for such diseases, as may be prescribed.
- A bank shall not supply the sperm or oocyte of a single donor to more than one commissioning couple.
- An oocyte donor shall be an ever married woman having at least one live child of her own with a minimum age of three years and to donate oocytes only once in her life and not more than seven oocyte shall be retrieved from the oocyte donor.
- All unused oocytes shall be preserved by the banks for use on the same recipient, or given for research to an organizations registered under this Act after seeking written consent from the commissioning couple.
- A bank shall obtain all necessary information in respect of a sperm or oocyte donor, including the name, identity and address of such donor, in such manner as may be prescribed, and shall undertake in writing from such donor about the confidentiality of such information.

1. Any medical geneticist, gynecologist, registered medical practitioner or any person, shall not:
   a. Abandon, disown or exploit or cause to be abandoned, disowned or exploited in any form the child or children born through ART;

b. Sell human embryo or gametes, run an agency, a racket or an organization for selling, purchasing or trading in human embryos or gametes;
c. Import or help in getting imported in whatsoever manner, the human embryos or human gametes;
d. Exploit the commissioning couple, woman or the gamete donor in any form;
e. Transfer human embryo into a male person or an animal;
f. Sell any human embryo or gamete for the purpose of research; or
g. Use any intermediates to obtain gamete donors or purchase gamete donors.

2. Whoever contravenes the provisions of clauses (a) to (g) of subsection (1), shall be punishable with a fine which shall not be less than five lakh rupees but may extend to ten lakh rupees for the first contravention and for subsequent contravention, shall be punishable with imprisonment for a term which shall not be less than eight years but may extend to twelve years and with fine which shall not be less than ten lakh rupees but may extend to twenty lakh rupees.
3. Whoever contravenes any of the provisions of this Act or any rules made thereunder, for which no penalty has been provided in this Act shall be punishable. All the offences under this Act shall be cognizable and bailable.

SUMMARY OF STATEMENT

Assisted reproductive technology has grown by leaps and bounds in the last few years. India has highest growths in the ART centers and the number of ART cycles performed every year. ART including IVF, has given hope to a multitude of persons suffering from infertility, but it has also introduced a plethora of legal, ethical and social issues. India has over the years become one of the major centers of this global fertility industry, with reproductive medical tourism becoming a significant activity. Clinics in India offer nearly all the ART services—gamete donation, intrauterine insemination (IUI), IVF, intracytoplasmic sperm injection (ICSI), preimplantation genetic diagnosis (PGD), and gestational surrogacy. However, in spite of so much activity in India, there is yet no standardization of protocols and reporting is still very inadequate. Furthermore, there is no law to regulate ART and it is regulated through guidelines.

The need to regulate the ART services is mainly to protect the affected women and children from exploitation. The oocyte donor needs to be supported by an insurance cover. Multiple embryo implantation needs to be regulated and children born through ART need to be protected. The cryopreservation of sperm, oocytes and embryo by the ART banks need to be regulated and the proposed legislation intends to make preimplantation genetic testing (PGT) mandatory for the benefit of the child born through ART.

There is a need to regulate ART clinics and banks by establishing the National Board, the State Boards, the National Registry and the State Registration Authorities for the regulation and supervision of ART clinics and the ART banks, for prevention of misuse and for safe and ethical practice of ART services.

The proposed legislation, namely, the ART (Regulation) Bill, 2020 proposes to regulate the ART services in the country. The salient features of the Bill are as follows:

a. To define certain terms like "ART", "ART clinic", "commissioning couple", "woman", etc.;
b. To provide that the National Board and the State Board shall be the same Board as proposed in the Surrogacy Bill;
c. To provide that the existing ART clinics and the ART banks, as on the date of the enactment of the proposed legislation, conducting ART procedures partly or exclusively shall make an application to the Registration Authority within a period of sixty days from the date of establishment of the National Registry;
d. To provide that the ART services shall be available to a woman above the legal age of marriage and below the age of 50 years and a man above the legal age of marriage and below the age of 55 years;
e. To provide that an oocyte donor shall be an ever married woman having at least one live child of her own with a minimum age of three years and to donate oocytes only once in her life and not more than seven oocyte shall be retrieved from the oocyte donor;
f. To provide that the ART clinics shall provide professional counseling to commissioning couple and woman about all the implications and and chances of success of ART procedures in the clinic; and they shall also inform the advantages, disadvantages and cost of the procedures, their medical side-effects, risks including the risk of multiple pregnancy and any such other matter as may help the commissioning couple to arrive at an informed decision that would most likely be the best for the commissioning couple and woman;
g. To provide that the ART clinics and ART banks shall ensure that commissioning couple, woman and donors of gametes are eligible to avail of ART procedures;
h. To provide for offences and penalties for the contravention of its provisions.
i. The notes on clauses explain in detail the various provisions contained in the Bill.
j. The Bill seeks to achieve the above objectives.

■ REFERENCE

1. The Assisted Reproductive Technology (Regulation) Bill, 2020. Bill no. 97 of 2020.

www.ingramcontent.com/pod-product-compliance
Ingram Content Group UK Ltd.
Pitfield, Milton Keynes, MK11 3LW, UK
UKHW052202140425
457402UK00003B/21